The Ethics Of Assisted Death

When Life Becomes A Burden Too Hard To Bear

Kenneth Cauthen

CSS Publishing Company, Inc., Lima, Ohio

THE ETHICS OF ASSISTED DEATH

Copyright © 1999 by
CSS Publishing Company, Inc.
Lima, Ohio

All rights reserved. No part of this publication may be reproduced in any manner whatsoever without the prior permission of the publisher, except in the case of brief quotations embodied in critical articles and reviews. Inquiries should be addressed to: Permissions, CSS Publishing Company, Inc., P.O. Box 4503, Lima, Ohio 45802-4503.

Library of Congress Cataloging-in-Publication Data

Cauthen, Kenneth, 1930-
 The ethics of assisted death : when life becomes a burden too hard to bear / Kenneth Cauthen.
     p. cm.
 ISBN 0-7880-1332-7 (pbk.)
 1. Assisted suicide—Moral and ethical aspects. I. Title.
R726.C385   1999
174'.24—dc21   98-44910
                                                                             CIP

ISBN 0-7880-1332-7   PRINTED IN U.S.A.

TO MY GRANDSON

Jacob Harllee Cauthen-Brown

Born: May 20, 1997

The first evidence of his superior intelligence was that he chose his parents wisely.

Table Of Contents

Preface	7
Chapter 1 Cases To Ponder: Initial Reflections	11
Chapter 2 The Problem And Some Proposals	25
Chapter 3 The Main Arguments: Against And For	41
Chapter 4 The Slippery-Slope Argument: The Logical Version	57
Chapter 5 The Slippery-Slope Argument: The Empirical Version	67
Chapter 6 The Heart Of the Debate: Two Difficult Issues	77
Chapter 7 Where We Are And A Suggestion	87
Suggestions For Further Reading	99

Preface

What are we to do when life becomes an intolerable burden rather than a cherished blessing? How are we to respond to others who find themselves in this grievous predicament with no hope of ever recovering health and the joy of living? Are we ever justified in choosing to die by deliberate action? Is it ever right to aid those who request assistance in dying? These questions are being widely debated today and will continue in the forefront of public discussion for many years to come. Many of us will confront these perplexing problems in our own lives or those of someone near and dear. My aim in this book is to give reasons for thinking that individuals should be given wide latitude in deciding when life should be ended by voluntary choice. Attitudes are changing, and I make the case for a change of law with respect to physician-assisted suicide and physician-administered death.

I write from a religious point of view, and I make explicit the biblical and philosophical foundations of my thinking. I offer these reflections not because I have all the right answers but to make a contribution to the ongoing debate. My reason for writing is to stimulate thinking and to provoke responses so that all of us may learn to think more profoundly about what love and mercy require when unbearable suffering for which there is no remedy has robbed life of its delight. I have learned much in the research and writing, but I do not harbor any illusions that I have resolved all the quandaries involved.

I have set forth my convictions as clearly and as honestly as I know how to do. I have also presented the views of those who take a position contrary to mine as fairly as I could. I have acknowledged the strengths of opposing opinions while giving reasons for preferring my own way of thinking. I believe that the reader will find here all the major ideas and attitudes that are currently being offered on both sides of the controversy. I invite evaluations and suggestions from those who support and from those who reject my point of view. My purpose will be fulfilled if all who enter the dialogue can come to a deeper understanding and achieve greater wisdom about these ultimate matters of life and death.

Not every issue important to the discussion is dealt with in this essay. I have concentrated on the arguments for and against assisted dying. Beyond that we should take note of the fact that attitudes vary with class, race, gender, and age. What is the significance of the fact that those who are most opposed to legalization of assisted death are African-Americans, those with low incomes, women, and people more than 75 years old? Those who are in favor tend to be white, middle or upper class, well-off economically, and well-educated, in other words, persons accustomed to having a lot of control over their lives. Neither do I explore the different perspectives that arise within Roman Catholic, Jewish, and Protestant traditions, not to mention other historic religions. I do not examine the various philosophical schools of thought for their insights and conflicting points of view. We come to our conclusions for many reasons rooted in our social and cultural location, life history and personal experience, family and religious background, intellectual training, personal reflection, and so on. Why we believe as we do is important and sometimes more interesting than what we believe. All of these topics are worthy of investigation. This small effort cannot do it all, but there is much to ponder in what is dealt with.

Many books and articles have been consulted in preparation for writing about this subject. This is the first book, however, for which most of the research has been done on the Internet. I found it a marvelous resource and discovered answers to questions more quickly and easily than I could have by using the excellent libraries nearby. This has made documentation more difficult or at least different from customary procedures. I have provided a list of recent books for those who would like to do further reading.

I have included far fewer endnotes than is conventional in a document of this type. Much of the information has come from the Internet and not from books. I have typically given references only when material is quoted or specific people are named. I have not given Internet addresses since they frequently change along with the content. Anyone who wants to use the Internet as a resource or to check out my claims can easily do so by using the standard search engines and typing in topics or names. Much useful material will be forthcoming.

Kenneth Cauthen
Rochester, New York
March 24, 1998

Chapter 1

Cases To Ponder: Initial Reflections

Debates on assisted death are based on principles of moral reasoning. They take place in the realm of theory. But the agonizing questions with their dilemmas full of conflicting values originate in actual life. It is in the experience of real people that the tragedies, ambiguities, and complexities that baffle thought are lived out. It is in their suffering and dying that the results of our legal and moral theories are put into practice. I begin with some well-known cases that have brought these life and death issues into the courts and into public discussion. Some of them represent important turning points in legal theory as well as in moral philosophy. Three of them brought forth landmark court decisions, two in the Supreme Court of the United States. First, the cases will be presented in factual and descriptive form, and then I will offer some commentary as a background to introducing the definitions, distinctions, principles, arguments, and proposals that occupy the rest of the essay. An examination of the eight cases to follow will raise the major questions having to do with the right to receive assistance in dying.

Dax Cowart

Dax Cowart was 25 years old in 1973 when he went with his father to look at a piece of land in Henderson, Texas. Afterward, when he tried to start his car, the ignition set off a huge accumulation of propane gas from a leaking underground pipe. He was badly burned over two-thirds of his body and suffered excruciating pain beyond anything he ever imagined possible. He begged a farmer to get a gun and kill him. The farmer replied, "I can't do that, son." Despite his protests, Mr. Cowart was taken to a local hospital and then to Dallas, where he pleaded for painkillers in the emergency room. Attendants insisted on asking him a lot of questions first. An IV was started, but it was six hours before he was given pain medicine. At every stage he asked not to be treated, but no one heeded him. However, his mother, Ada, and the family lawyer, Rex Houston, urged that treatment continue without pause.

For fourteen months he was subjected to almost daily immersions, sometimes twice a day, using bleach to care for his wounds and remove dead tissue. He described these repeated baths that exposed bare muscle and bone as painful beyond words to describe. Many times great arguments ensued as he protested what was being done to him. He physically resisted doctors and nurses to the extent that his limited physical abilities permitted, but to no avail. A psychiatrist who was called in to examine his mental state declared him to be competent to make decisions. Nevertheless, the treatments continued even though he continued to plead that they be stopped. He asked for help in dying. Since he had lost use of his hands, he could not kill himself but made several unsuccessful efforts.

After many months he was transferred to Houston Medical Center and then weeks later to John Sealey Hospital in Galveston. Despite his continued protests, he went through more treatments, including surgery on his arms and hands as well as skin grafts. He was completely blind, severely deaf, and had no fingers and only part of one thumb. Most of his ears were gone, and he was severely disfigured. Eventually, he was discharged from the hospital, later married, went to law school, and began a successful practice. He became a passionate advocate of patients' rights and gave lectures on his horrible experiences. He admits to achieving a level of happiness he didn't believe possible. While he is glad to be alive, Mr. Cowart still thinks he should have been allowed to die and that he should not have been treated without his consent. He insists that no one had the right to put him through the hell he endured.

Karen Ann Quinlan

Karen Ann Quinlan of New Jersey was 21 years old when on April 14, 1975, at a party she took some drugs and drank alcohol at a bar. She dozed off, and when she could not be revived was taken to an emergency room but never regained consciousness. Eventually she moved into what physicians called a chronic persistent vegetative state. Ms. Quinlan was unable to breathe without a mechanical respirator and unable to eat without a feeding tube. She had no cognitive functions and would, in the opinion of doctors, never recover. After some months, her parents petitioned the courts in New Jersey to have the respirator disconnected with the expectation that she would die. Priests assured her Roman Catholic family that it was morally permissible to permit her to die. A superior court ruled that the respirator could not be shut off, but the New Jersey Supreme Court reversed that judgment and gave permission for the respirator to be removed. Nuns in charge of her care, anticipating this decision but opposed to it, had been gradually reducing the time she was on the respirator. When it was removed, Ms. Quinlan did not die. Her parents did not request that the feeding tube be removed, and it was not. She remained, however, in the persistent vegetative state, reduced to skin and bones. She lived for ten more years and died in June 1985.

Elizabeth Bouvia

Elizabeth Bouvia entered a hospital in Riverside, California, in September of 1983. She was a 26-year-old woman with cerebral palsy. Her desire was to die of starvation but she wanted painkillers to keep her comfortable. Given her condition, she said this was the only way she could commit suicide. The hospital declined the request, and the case went to court. She was turned down by the trial court, but on April 16, 1986, the California Court of Appeals, Second District, overturned the ruling of the lower court. The court ordered that the feeding tube be removed and that no one could put it back without her consent. The tube had been inserted against her will and contrary to her written instructions. The Court noted that she was quadriplegic, could only move some of her fingers on one hand, and make slight movements of her face and head. She was totally dependent on others for everything. After she gained the right to die, Ms. Bouvia changed her mind. She began to eat voluntarily and indicated that she would try to get better. Ms. Bouvia was still alive ten years later. In an interview in 1997 shown on television, she said that she was in great agony after the tube was removed and agreed to its replacement. She did say, however, that she still wished she were dead.

Nancy Cruzan

On January 11, 1983, Nancy Cruzan lost control of her car in Jasper County, Missouri, and was severely injured. Heart and lung functions were restored, but oxygen deprivation had irreparably damaged her brain. She was in a deep coma for three weeks and eventually moved into a permanent vegetative state. She showed no cognitive function and could not swallow. A feeding tube was put in her stomach. After some time in which she showed no improvement, her family decided that this was not a way that Nancy would want to exist and asked the hospital staff to remove the feeding tube. The request was denied. The family took the case to a state court and was granted an order to have the tube removed. A friend testified that Ms. Cruzan had once told her that she would not want to live in that condition. The state of Missouri, however, appealed the case because of the uncertainty as to whether the court order demonstrably reflected Nancy's wishes. The case finally went to the Supreme Court of the United States. A split decision was rendered in 1990 which recognized the right of a patient to refuse medical treatment. The Court concluded, however, that the state of Missouri was not wrong in requiring clear and convincing evidence that Nancy would ask to die if she were competent to decide. The case was sent back to Missouri for a final decision. This time several friends came forward to confirm that Nancy had clearly let it be known that she would rather die than live like this. Nancy's doctor, who had originally opposed the removal of the tube, testified that it would be in her best interest to die. The court was convinced and ordered the removal of the tube. She died on December 26, 1990, after eleven days of dehydration and starvation.

Sue Rodriguez

Sue Rodriguez of Canada was forty years old when she was diagnosed with ALS (amyotrophic lateral sclerosis, also known as

Lou Gehrig's disease). She knew that death was not far away and that eventually she would lose her ability to walk, move her body, eat, and breathe without assistance. Preferring not to live this way, she wanted means provided so that by her own actions she could end her life. She wanted a physician present in case something went wrong. She took her case to the courts, getting a negative response in December 1992. The Chief Justice of the British Columbia Court of Appeals in May 1993 decided that she did have a right to request a physician to assist her in committing suicide, but two other Justices ruled against her. The case went to the Supreme Court of Canada, and in September 1993 the Justices voted against her five to four, although all nine agreed that the present law infringed on her rights as a person. It is certain that she was assisted to die on February 12, 1994, since she was not physically able to do what was necessary by herself. The cause of death was respiratory failure due to the presence of drugs in her body. It was established that Svend Robinson was present, and perhaps someone else, maybe a physician, but the evidence was insufficient to bring charges against Robinson for aiding Ms. Rodriguez to die.

Austin Bastable

In September 1995, three years after Sue Rodriguez first sought assistance in dying, Austin Bastable, a citizen of Ontario, Canada, gave a press conference. He laid out the steps he had been taking to get public support for a change in the law so that people like himself and Ms. Rodriguez could legally be assisted to die at their request. A former tool-and-die maker, he had been suffering from progressive multiple sclerosis for 26 years, approximately half his life. He indicated that while he received loving care from his wife and family, he suffered greatly every day. Mr. Bastable had made an unsuccessful attempt to commit suicide in November 1994. That convinced him that without aid he could not end his life. He wanted the opportunity to choose the time of his death and to have assistance in ways that would not lead to charges of murder against those who helped him. Mr. Bastable said specifically that he did not want to die by just any means but sought help in accordance with the highest legal, ethical, and medical standards available. He made it clear, however, that he would find a way in accordance with his own wishes. Mr. Bastable expressed regret that he had to spend his last days trying to change unjust laws and plunging himself into controversy. He did it, he said, out of conviction and for the sake of other suffering Canadians like himself who were too ill, too weak, or too afraid to speak out. When his intentions came into public view, opponents of the right to choose death instituted a movement to save him. A supporter noted that he was bombarded with so much "Christian love" from his would-be saviors that his e-mail system had to be shut down. He observed that they only made "Austin's life even more miserable than it already was." Mr. Bastable died May 6, 1996, with the assistance of Dr. Jack Kevorkian.

Robert Latimer

On October 24, 1993, in Saskatchewan, Canada, Robert Latimer reported to police that his twelve-year-old daughter had died in her sleep. He was at home alone with Tracy while his wife and their other children were at church. The coroner, after an autopsy, indicated that her blood contained a deadly level of carbon monoxide. Latimer, a wheat and canola farmer, then confessed that he had put his daughter in his pickup truck and pumped exhaust fumes into the cabin until she died. Afterward he took Tracy back in the house and put her in bed. She had suffered from cerebral palsy all her life. She weighed less than forty pounds and could not walk, talk, or feed herself. Tracy had undergone numerous operations on her back, hips, and legs. She experienced a great deal of discomfort and suffered from repeated seizures. In late 1993 another major operation on her hip had been scheduled. The purpose was to stabilize metal rods that had been placed in her back a year earlier so that she could stay upright. Doctors also planned to insert a feeding tube because the anti-seizure medicine caused problems for her appetite and digestion. Her parents feared that she faced a life of constant pain. Laura, her mother, said she did not have the courage to do what her husband did but agreed that it was best for Tracy.

A jury found Mr. Latimer guilty of second-degree murder, and the judge imposed the mandatory sentence of life in prison with no eligibility for parole for ten years. The Supreme Court of Canada ordered a new trial because prosecutors had privately interviewed prospective jurors about their views on abortion and mercy-killing. Five of them ended up on the jury. In October 1997 a new trial began, and Latimer was again found guilty of second-degree murder. The jury, however, recommended parole after one year. On December 1, 1997, the judge agreed with the jury and granted a rare constitutional exemption. Judge Ted Noble ruled that the mandatory sentence of life imprisonment with no possibility of parole for ten years would be cruel and unusual punishment. Latimer was sentenced instead to serve one year in prison and a second year confined to his farm.

During the trial the prosecution called witnesses who testified that Tracy was a smiling, lovable child who was no worse off than many other disabled children. Her pain was said to be intermittent and situational. A journal written by Laura Latimer was introduced in which she described her daughter as alert and happy. Advocates of the disabled were alarmed at the widespread and deep sympathy shown to Robert Latimer, whom they saw as a murderer who deserved full punishment. All disabled people, they felt, are at risk in a society that puts so little value on people like Tracy. One opponent of the judge's decision declared, "It's a sick world when killing is called compassionate and punishment for killers is called cruel."

After her husband had been convicted at his first trial, Laura Latimer gave an emotionally-charged condemnation of the verdict. She defended him as a kind and loving father who did what was best for Tracy. She reviewed the life of pain and agony their daughter had lived. She told of the seizures Tracy suffered "every minute, every day for months" beginning when she was less than a year old. She spoke of the many painful operations Tracy underwent. Mrs. Latimer accused those who wanted her husband to spend the rest of his life in jail of being indifferent to the hell their daughter went through. She said the only thing that kept them going was thinking about Tracy. Mr. Latimer received thousands of letters of support commending him for being a loving father who relieved his daughter of a life of misery. His oldest half-brother commented that "it was unfortunate that this could not have been handled some other way."

Jane Doe

Jane Doe (not her real name) was a 76-year-old retired physical education instructor who lived in Oceanside, New York. She was one of the plaintiffs in a New York case that eventually went to the Supreme Court of the United States. She was a mentally competent, terminally-ill patient dying of thyroid cancer. Doctors told her recovery was impossible. A feeding tube was implanted that caused serious problems. She faced a dilemma between having her pain reduced to a tolerable level and remaining mentally alert. In her plea to the court she said, "At the point at which I can no longer endure the pain and suffering associated with my cancer, I want to have drugs available for the purpose of hastening my death in a humane and certain manner." In New York physician-assisted suicide is a criminal offense. Along with others she petitioned the courts to have this law declared unconstitutional. In April 1996 the Second Circuit Court in *Quill v. Vacco* concluded that New York's prohibition of assisted suicide is a violation of the Equal Protection provision of the Constitution. On June 26, 1997, the Supreme Court of the United States reversed that decision, stating that the Constitution upholds the right of a state to forbid assisted suicide. The unanimous verdict was that the Constitution does not guarantee a right to physician-assisted suicide, although states are free to permit or forbid it. By that time Jane Doe had died.

Some Initial Reflections

Death by choice has been discussed by philosophers and others for many centuries, but in the last half-century the issue has taken on new significance. In the 1950s developments in medical technology made it possible to keep some patients alive longer than ever before. In previous times terminally-ill and permanently unconscious patients who were unable to breathe and eat on their own would simply have died. Mechanical ventilators and artificial feeding tubes now enabled patients to get oxygen, fluids, and nutrition. It was not long before it became necessary for patients or their families to make decisions about how long life should be preserved. New and difficult moral questions arose.

Karen Ann Quinlan and Nancy Cruzan are mentioned in every textbook on bioethics. Their cases represent major turning points in theory and practice. The issue in both cases involves the right of patients or their proxies to refuse or to demand withdrawal of life-sustaining treatment. That right is now firmly established, but as recently as the 1970s it was not. The experience of Dax Cowart is vivid and horrifying evidence of this. A ventilator was removed from Ms. Quinlan, and a feeding tube was taken from Ms. Cruzan. Ms. Quinlan's father was asked whether he wanted his daughter's feeding tube removed, and he said, "Oh no, that is her nourishment." At one time a distinction was made between ventilators that provide oxygen and feeding tubes that provide hydration and nutrition. It was thought that ventilators could be shut off, but water and food had to be provided. Now that distinction has been abandoned. In practice today it is quite permissible upon legitimate request to withdraw any kind of life-sustaining treatment.

The issue now lies at a different point. Once treatment has been withdrawn in hopeless cases, must we let patients die over time as nature takes its course while only comfort care is provided? Or is it permissible, or in some cases mandatory, to provide a lethal injection that brings about a quick, easy death? Currently, only the first option is available. Deliberately to bring about a patient's death is considered to be murder. Letting die when patients are hopelessly ill and near death or permanently unconscious is one thing. Causing to die is quite another in current practice. But is this distinction morally defensible? Elizabeth Bouvia got a court order to have her feeding tube removed, but she found the process of starving so excruciating that she changed her mind. If Ms. Bouvia had requested it, would it have been morally permissible not only to remove her feeding tube but also to have a physician administer a lethal injection to cause the death for which she so fervently wished?

Elizabeth Bouvia was neither terminally ill nor unconscious. She did, however, require a feeding tube to keep her alive. She won the right to have the feeding tube removed, and had she gone through with it, she would have died. Another set of problems is raised by the cases of Sue Rodriguez and Austin Bastable. What the three of them had in common was a degenerative disease that robbed them of capacities they thought were essential to a life worth living. Each concluded that given the future that lay ahead, death was preferable to continuing to exist in the desperate condition in which they found themselves. Ms. Bouvia was still alive in 1997 but said then that she still wished she were dead. Rodriguez and Bastable found someone to help them die in ways that would not result in jail terms for their benefactors. All three were conscious, mentally-competent persons suffering from serious disabilities but were not near death. Unlike Ms. Bouvia, however, Ms. Rodriguez and Mr. Bastable did not require life-sustaining treatment that they could ask to have removed so that they could die. Does an individual in the situation of Austin Bastable and Sue Rodriguez have a right to receive assistance in dying if she or he decides that life is an intolerable burden worse than death?

The case of Dax Cowart poses still another set of problems. No other situation presented here, except that of Robert Latimer, rips the emotions and challenges the mind like this one. Mr. Cowart begged to die because the therapy he needed to save his life was so acutely painful that he preferred death to enduring it. In 1973 the right to refuse treatment was not yet established, and he was treated despite his unending, vehement protest. Nevertheless, he survived and in 1997 was still alive and enjoying a quality of life he was glad to have. Were the doctors and his mother right in coercing him against his will to endure the terrible and overwhelming torment he underwent on a daily basis for months on end? Mr. Cowart thought they were wrong and passionately insisted a quarter of a century later that he should have been allowed to die or even aided to die to relieve him of his intense suffering. Should his judgment be the last word on the subject? At the time it was not certain that he would survive with or without treatment. Who has the right to say to him that he was wrong when he and he alone had to experience the daily agony of extreme pain? Should he have been the judge then of whether death was preferable to his long ordeal?

Some people looking back are glad they did not have the option of choosing death when they were suffering greatly, since they are now alive and better. On a CBC broadcast in Canada on June 14, 1995, Dr. Arnold Voth told of treating a 75-year-old man with severe intestinal bleeding and serious heart problems. He spent two weeks in the hospital and went into a coma twice. For a week he begged the doctor daily in no uncertain terms to help him die. He recovered sufficiently to go home but later returned and once again asked to be killed. After that he returned from time to time for additional therapy. Two years later he was back, seriously ill, but this time requested a heart transplant since he had so much to live for.

On the same program Mark Pickup, a 42-year-old man with chronic progressive multiple sclerosis since 1984, told of his disabilities that made life a terrible burden. He reported that in 1985-86 his pain was so bad and he was so depressed and experiencing such deep sorrow and grief that, had he had the right to choose assistance in ending his life, he probably would have. Now he is glad to be alive and opposes the right of people like him to choose death. We can applaud the testimony of Mr. Pickup and honor the experience of Dr. Voth's patient. We can rejoice with them in their triumph and at the same time understand the witness of Dax Cowart. Sometimes values are in conflict. It is impossible to weigh them precisely in every case or to make universal judgments that have absolute validity.

Is it possible that different interpretations of the same situation could be equally right? Mr. Cowart knows he would have been dead years ago if his wishes had been granted, but he says that is all right. How can we say he is wrong? Mr. Pickup and Dr. Voth's elderly patient would likely have been dead also if the option of assisted death had been available. They are now glad it was not. We can hardly say they are wrong. We have ambiguous and tragic situations in which no answer can be right for everybody or which do not involve great suffering or an unnecessarily early death. Either way gains and losses are inseparable, and an unambiguously correct solution may not be possible. Obviously, some benefits are worth enduring much suffering for if they can be had no other way.

Yet at some point are the extent and duration of suffering so great that they justify an earlier death even if the person might eventually survive?

The cases of Dax Cowart and Robert Latimer are much more ambiguous and heartbreaking and the answers much less clear than in all the previous ones surveyed. Several features of the mercy killing involving Mr. Latimer are troubling. First of all, the consequences of his actions fell not on him alone but even more on his daughter. He made a choice for Tracy, who at twelve years of age had some understanding of her situation and of her future prospects. Only she experienced directly the pain and suffering of her disease. Tracy could not talk, and no reports that I have seen indicate whether Robert Latimer had any notion about her own wishes. Did she prefer to die rather than face a life of constant pain and suffering? Yet to ask her puts a burden on a child that was perhaps more than she should have been asked to bear. A twelve-year-old child is neither a mature adult nor an infant who has no understanding of what is going on. Conscious, competent adults can make the choice to live or die for themselves. Parents of necessity have to decide for their infant children. Where does Tracy Latimer fit? Children can sometimes rise to a level of understanding, acceptance, and maturity that not many adults ever attain.

It is a perplexing and troubling situation with no good solution. Some opponents accused him of relieving his own burden rather than his daughter's. But surely we can feel compassion for him and sympathize with the dilemma he faced. At the same time what he did was alarming and distressing and perhaps unwise and wrong. Human judgment is fallible in a situation like this, and reason is impotent. Even though he acted as a kind and caring father who did what he thought was best for the child he dearly loved, we still shudder to think about what he did. It was a mercy killing, and both terms have to be acknowledged without weakening either one. The legal system has no satisfactory remedy. Mr. Latimer is not a menace to society, and he has paid a heavy penalty already. Yet he did kill a child, and the law demands punishment. Neither setting him free nor sending him to prison is suitable. Unfortunately, society has been divided into angry camps, each accusing the other of being heartless and insensitive. No one is happy about the outcome. The most important question may not be how to punish him appropriately but how to salvage his life and that of his wife and living children. Beyond that, the whole community needs some way of coming to terms with this event that police, lawyers, judges, and juries cannot provide. We need ways of dealing with mercy killings that are reconciling and healing. We long for some way of providing saving discipline for Mr. Latimer and some means of attaining resolution and peace for us all in cases of tragic ambiguity like this. Ideally, religious communities provide the setting in which reflection, reconciliation, and redemption can take place. Many times and in manifold ways they do. Yet religion often exacerbates the problem by disputes over what God has to say about the situation.

The case of Jane Doe defines where the center of debate is at the moment. The Supreme Court decision of 1997 found no right to physician-assisted suicide in the Constitution but left the door open for states to permit it or forbid it. On November 4, 1997, the citizens of Oregon voted to keep their law allowing physician-assisted suicide. Jane Doe exemplifies exactly the circumstances in which the strongest possible case can be made in favor. She was an elderly, competent, fully-informed, terminally-ill patient near death experiencing intolerable pain and suffering that could not be relieved without compromising her mental alertness. She was not asking that a physician administer drugs that would kill her, but only that her doctor be allowed to make available medicines that she could take by her own action if she decided that death was preferable to living a little longer. Should physician-assisted suicide defined in this way be made legal? This question defines the heart of the controversy going on right now.

In conclusion, let me make a point that will bear repeating throughout. Many of the issues with which we must deal confront us with irresolvable contradictions in which good and bad are inseparably intertwined. Moral and societal remedies are not fully adequate. Human choice and action cannot escape or transcend the ambiguities that baffle us. Only a religious resolution will suffice.

Our final appeal is to the grace of a loving God who knows, cares, and understands the insoluble dilemmas we face in this life. Our only hope is to find solace in the arms of a Caring Companion who suffers with us and who accepts us without condemnation when we do the best we can in situations in which it is not possible to do good without at the same time doing harm (Matthew 13:24-30; Psalm 103).

In the next chapter I will offer some definitions, make some distinctions, and set forth my own convictions about the rights of individuals to request assistance in dying. I will also outline the theological and ethical presuppositions that guide my thinking.

Chapter 2

The Problem And Some Proposals

Life is a precious gift to be received from the Creator with gratitude. It should be cherished, preserved, and enhanced in every way possible. But when the potential for meaningful, joyful, desirable life has been thoroughly exhausted and every effort made to prevent the inevitable, we should make it legally possible for the merciful to show mercy to the dying who request intervention to end their suffering.

The only appropriate way to make this claim is with deep humility and in fear and trembling. We must always stand in awe and reverence when life itself is at stake. As Dr. Timothy Quill has said, anyone who thinks this question has a simple or obvious answer has not thought very deeply or seriously about the matter. Those who are opposed to making it legal for physicians to provide aid in dying make arguments and voice fears that are formidable indeed. Nevertheless, I conclude that the stronger case would legally permit physicians under carefully regulated conditions to provide assistance in dying for those who request it.

Before we proceed, it is necessary to offer some definitions and make some distinctions that will aid us in knowing precisely what we are talking about.

Definitions And Distinctions

Passive Euthanasia[1]: The termination of life-sustaining treatment by a doctor, nurse, technician, or someone else, with the informed consent of the patient or of authorized proxies when the patient is comatose or incompetent. It can refer also to the withholding of life-sustaining treatment in hopeless cases.

Active Euthanasia: The deliberate ending of life by a physician or someone else in order to bring about a good or desired death. It usually refers to the administration of medicines by a medical professional that intentionally cause death based on the full, informed consent of patients or their authorized proxies.

Voluntary **Active Euthanasia**: Active euthanasia in which a fully-informed patient is competent to make the decision and does so.

Non-voluntary **Active Euthanasia**: Active euthanasia in which the patient is in a coma or otherwise incompetent to decide and the decision is made by family or other persons qualified to do so.[2]

Involuntary **Active Euthanasia**: Active euthanasia without the consent of the patient. The person is capable of giving informed consent but refuses to do so or is not asked. This is murder and can never be justified. No one in the current debate argues for killing a person who wants to live, regardless of the suffering he or she is undergoing.

Mercy Killing refers either to voluntary active euthanasia or to non-voluntary active euthanasia.[3]

Physician-Assisted Suicide: The provision of medications or procedures by a doctor that a patient can use to commit suicide. The death-bringing act itself is performed by the person desiring to die by using the means provided. Non-physicians also may provide means that someone may use to commit suicide.

Physician-Administered Death: The administration of medicines that cause death upon request of the patient or a proxy. This is a form of active euthanasia. Non-physicians may also upon request take measures out of compassion that actually end the life of another and thus engage in a type of active euthanasia that we sometimes call mercy killing.

Not everyone uses exactly these full terms in every case, but it is usually clear from the context which of these procedures is meant. Some definitions overlap others. The following scheme outlines the main positions taken today. While various subgroups might be formed within each group, in some cases involving overlapping between the major groups, these are the major points of division.[4]

GROUP 1

Approve

Passive Euthanasia

Oppose

All forms of Assisted Suicide and all forms of Active Euthanasia

GROUP 2

Passive Euthanasia
Physician-Assisted Suicide
Non-Physician-Assisted Suicide

All forms of Active Euthanasia

GROUP 3

Passive Euthanasia
Assisted Suicide
   Physician-Assisted Suicide
   Non-Physician-Assisted Suicide
Active Euthanasia
   Physician-Administered Death
   Mercy Killing

Involuntary Active Euthanasia

Group 1 allows only the possibility of withholding or removing life-sustaining equipment, assuming a voluntary request by the patient or authorized proxy. Passive euthanasia merely allows nature to take its course by recognizing the limits of medical science. But it is impermissible to assist another person actively to commit suicide or to take the life of another intentionally, even if requested to do so.

Group 2 would go a step further and also permit doctors to provide the means for people to end their lives under carefully restricted conditions. They might not permit non-physicians to assist in the suicide of another outside a legally regulated setting. Others might in some cases justify non-physician-assisted suicide in an informal context. All in this group would draw a bright line between permitted forms of assisted suicide and all forms of active euthanasia.

Group 3 goes still further and adds various forms of active euthanasia. In particular, this group approves physician-administered death under carefully regulated and restricted conditions. Some might forbid all non-physician forms of assisted suicide and administered death outside a carefully monitored setting. Others would want to make a judgment about non-physician forms of assisted suicide and administered death on a case by case basis. Mercy killing may involve non-voluntary active euthanasia. That makes it even more necessary to examine particular instances, since some may not be justified. Involuntary active euthanasia is forbidden in all cases.

Everyone would insist on defining exactly the circumstances under which each of the approved procedures could actually be employed in accordance with ethical principles. Not every instance in a category would necessarily meet all the essential criteria to make it a legitimate moral act. The categories that are opposed are forbidden under all circumstances. The categories that are approved indicate a class of actions that in principle might be moral but only if certain conditions are met. Those in Group 3, for example, would not necessarily approve every instance of active euthanasia, even upon the request of a patient or proxies.

These classifications are designed to reflect what various people regard as morally right or wrong. A further question arises as to which of the morally-approved activities should also be made legal. Currently active euthanasia is against the law everywhere, although the legal practice of giving heavy doses of pain medicine with the intent of relieving suffering even though it hastens death comes close. Terminal sedation, which puts patients into a deep anesthetized sleep as a last resort to relieve pain until they die, comes even closer to qualifying as active euthanasia.

In what follows I take a position within Group 3. However, the focus of attention is on the role of physicians in assisting patients to end their lives or in administering medicines that cause their death. Some ambiguity with regard to the usage of terms is unavoidable given the way the discussion is carried on today. Strictly speaking, physician-assisted suicide refers only to the provision of means that a patient can use to commit suicide. I will speak of physician-assisted dying to include either or both physician-assisted suicide and physician-administered death (active euthanasia). As the presentation unfolds, it should be evident what is intended in each instance, so that no confusion should result from these complexities.

Morally, no difference exists between physician-assisted suicide and physician-administered death, in my view. Physicians, patients, and their families may feel differently about the two and find assisted suicide easier to accept than active euthanasia. But the morality depends on the conditions under which the patient's life is ended and whether or not fully informed consent is given. Ethical rightness does not turn on whether the physician merely puts lethal medicine at the bedside to be used by a patient by choice or whether the physician injects lethal medicine upon legitimate request of a competent person or proxy. Physician-assisted suicide may be preferred when that is possible, but it is not morally superior to physician-administered death when the required conditions are met. Furthermore, to limit assistance to providing lethal medicine that a person may use discriminates against those who are not physically capable of swallowing a pill or activating a device that ends their lives.

In my opinion, a persuasive case for physician-assisted dying can be made in two types of cases: the terminally ill and the permanently unconscious. A third category should not be ruled out: when death is better than life. A fourth classification is problematic and dangerous but in some cases may be justifiable: mercy killing. Each requires elaboration.

The Terminally Ill: The strongest case for physician-assisted suicide and physician-administered death can be made for those who have not much life left no matter what we do, and their condition is such that dying sooner rather than later is preferable. Jane Doe is an example of this circumstance. Four conditions are required:

    1. The patient is dying, and no remedy is available.

    2. The patient is in unbearable, unmanageable pain or suffering beyond the power of present medical science to alleviate.

3. The patient is fully informed, mentally competent, and makes a voluntary request for assistance in dying.

4. The choice of death is an enduring one after thorough reflection and due consideration of all alternatives and future possibilities.

The Permanently Unconscious: An equally strong case can be made for physician-assisted death for those who have no hope of ever attaining consciousness again. In these cases, physical life continues at some level, but the capacities essential to personhood are beyond recovery. The patient in an irreversible coma is unable to speak or to recognize or respond to family and friends. No communication is possible, and the patient is unaware of self or others. Karen Ann Quinlan and Nancy Cruzan are examples. Doctors declared both of them to be in a persistent vegetative state. In instances of this sort, it is in no one's interest to keep the patient alive. All that made life worthwhile has disappeared and cannot be recovered. It does not matter to the person one way or another, since there is no consciousness of anything. This way of existence is the same as being dead as far as the patient is concerned. The family can see and touch a body that has a beating heart, but the person they knew and loved is gone forever. No compelling reason or purpose can be given for keeping a body alive when the person is effectively already dead. On the basis of the patient's previously stated wishes or with the consent of authorized proxies, the life-sustaining equipment can be removed. If that is done, it should also be permissible and in some cases mandatory to give a lethal injection to ensure a quick and easy death.

When Death Is Better Than Life: Beyond these two types of cases, two others arise that are more ambiguous. A strong argument can be made that Elizabeth Bouvia, Sue Rodriguez, and Austin Bastable qualify for physician-assisted suicide or physician-administered death (voluntary active euthanasia). Some people have progressive degenerative diseases that gradually take away all their capacities to care for themselves, to work, and to enjoy life. Or they may be so totally paralyzed or otherwise disabled or afflicted that for them no meaning or purpose justifies the effort to stay alive. Pain and suffering may make daily life an agonizing ordeal so that the limits of endurance are reached. With no hope of cure and a prospect of nothing ahead but greater degeneration and increasing suffering, a person may decide that death would be better than the continuation of what has become an unendurable existence. Life has become so wretched as not to be worth preserving, since all that made life good has forever disappeared. Once it has been determined that the choice to die is enduring, voluntary, and made in full consciousness of the meaning and consequences of the act, it is permissible to cease life-sustaining treatment. It is also permissible for a physician to administer lethal medicines that will terminate life as quickly and humanely as possible. Physician-administered death is especially needed if the patient is not physically able to swallow medicines or activate a device that will end his or her life.

This must, of course, be an individual, voluntary choice. No person can decide for another when life has ceased to be worthwhile. We should allow people to make that decision for themselves and honor it when it reflects an enduring conclusion duly made after consideration of all alternatives and consequences. Any determination should include their responsibilities and connections to other people who will be affected. This decision must not be forced on anyone. No pressure whatsoever must be exerted to persuade or lead anyone to this choice. Finally, every effort humanly and societally possible must be made in every instance to create situations for suffering people that make continuing to live preferable to dying by choice.

The example of Stephen Hawking is wondrously inspiring in this regard.[5] Although motor neuron disease (also called ALS or Lou Gehrig's disease) has progressively robbed him of many physical capacities, his brilliant mind continues to function at the highest level. He is one of the giants of twentieth-century science. We rejoice in his mental triumph over bodily tragedy. It is marvelous that he has been able to find life worthwhile, challenging, and full of joy despite his disabilities, and he graces it all with a sense of humor. What his ultimate destiny and choice will be, we cannot say in 1998, but whatever choice he makes now and in the future is his alone to make and should be honored.

Each case must be taken on its own. Elizabeth Bouvia, Sue Rodriguez, and Austin Bastable should have their choices respected and heeded. Dax Cowart is still alive but has never relented in his insistence that he should have been allowed to die. I do not see how anyone can claim to know better than he what should have been done. It is after all his life and his suffering that are in question, and no one doubts his mental competence to understand the issues and to make an informed choice.

Mercy Killing: A fourth category is even more difficult, and generalizations are hazardous. Mercy killings are problematic and raise serious questions. I would not absolutely rule them out but would insist on making a case by case judgment. Some instances are heartbreaking and tragic. The case of Robert Latimer is an example of the baffling issues raised by mercy killing. We may be at a loss to know whether to approve or not. Given the fact that assistance in dying is against the law, we put people in absolutely intolerable situations in some tormenting circumstances. They are faced with watching a loved one suffer great pain and agony that cannot be relieved without their committing murder. It is most sorrowful when the suffering victim begs to be killed. The most troubling and ambiguous are instances of non-voluntary active euthanasia in which the person is incompetent because of age or mental disability or when the wishes of the person whose life is ended are unknown.

One can, of course, imagine an extreme situation in which even the voluntary principle would not necessarily hold, if it requires an explicit request. Suppose a person were trapped in a burning car with absolutely no possibility either of being rescued or of surviving. Suppose further that the person is conscious and in torment but cannot communicate his or her wishes. Would it be permissible to kill that person immediately with a gun, if one were available? In some drastic circumstances like this, it would be immoral not to violate the voluntary principle. To invoke the Golden Rule, I would earnestly hope that if I were in that situation, some kind soul would do the dreadful deed to relieve me of useless agony. Nevertheless, except for these fortunately rare circumstances at the furthest margins of life, the principle that a request must be made voluntarily by a competent person or appropriate proxies is inviolable.

Involuntary active euthanasia, however, is murder and is absolutely forbidden under all circumstances. No person should ever be killed contrary to his or her wish. No one in the current debate has endorsed ending the life of a person who explicitly objects. That is the absolute line that must never be crossed.

Two remedies are available to lessen the anguish of mercy killing. (1) Assistance in dying should be legalized under carefully regulated conditions. This would eliminate the necessity of mercy killings in many if not most instances. (2) Beyond that I agree with James Rachels[6] that mercy killing should be made into a legal defense of killing in the same way that self-defense now is. If a perpetrator can show that the killing was justified under the circumstances and was done out of mercy to relieve intolerable suffering when no other remedy was available, the accused could be acquitted by a jury.

A Defense Of My Proposals

Let me pause here to acknowledge that some will find some of my proposals appalling. In particular some disabled persons and their advocates react with terror and horror at the suggestion that people might be deliberately killed to relieve their suffering. They are fearful that people with disabilities would be at great risk if my recommendations became lawful. Permitting active euthanasia suggests to many that people with disabilities have no value and therefore can be eliminated for the convenience of society or to save money. I fully understand and appreciate these feelings, although I take a different point of view. I can only say that I have come to my conclusions out of compassion for suffering people in the light of the best wisdom available to me. I defend my proposals because the alternatives are even worse. Whether I am right or not, my only motivations are love and mercy for people at the extremes of life who face dreadful options. My argument is simply that **in some circumstances, putting an end to suffering may take priority over extending life.** A great deal depends on whether that principle is accepted or not. The discussion over the rightness of assisted suicide and administered death should not turn on whether some people are heartless, insensitive, and cruel in comparison with others, but on what love, mercy, and compassion permit or require in these heartbreaking, tormenting situations at the extremes of life that we all wish we could avoid.

Killing and suicide are words that have strong negative connotations and provoke a powerful emotional response. If some are horrified at the notion that sometimes it is permissible deliberately to end the life of a person who requests it or who is permanently unconscious, I am horrified at the thought of forcing people to endure awful suffering when they are begging to die. How much torment are we willing to impose on people against their will to quiet our deeply-ingrained qualms regarding suicide or killing?

Here is what I have proposed:

1. That dying patients undergoing intolerable agony that medical science cannot relieve be legally assisted to die if they request it. Why should we force people hopelessly at death's door to suffer unnecessarily and pointlessly when they themselves prefer to die?

2. That patients in a permanent coma with no hope of recovery be legally assisted to die on the basis of their previously expressed wishes or at the request of their authorized proxies. Why should we keep patients alive who have no awareness of themselves or others and who will never again exist as the conscious, precious persons they once were?

3. That some persons whose lives are experienced by them as worse than death should be allowed upon their request to have assistance in dying in a humane and lawful way. Why should we force people whose lives are an unbearable burden to endure suffering, perhaps for many years, against their own enduring choice, judgment, and will?

4. That sometimes in rare, extreme, desperate circumstances a person may be morally justified in killing another out of mercy to relieve suffering. Is it never permissible to end the life of another no matter how awful or hopeless that life has become, even if the person living that life begs to die?

I readily admit that all of these proposals have risks, difficulties, problems, and dangers that cannot be avoided. I concede that abuses are possible and that mistakes might be made. I maintain only that the alternatives are less satisfactory when everything is taken into account. Worse abuses are possible and actually occur now than would happen if my recommendations were accepted, or so I believe.

Theological And Ethical Assumptions

I write as a Protestant theologian. Every moral affirmation in this book presupposes a set of theological premises that come from the specific religious tradition in which I stand. In addition, I make some ethical and value presuppositions based on experience interpreted by reason. While the distinction between Scripture and reason is useful for some purposes, it is somewhat artificial and of limited validity, at least in my case. Each source of insight is interpreted through the other to produce a unified body of convictions that function as a whole. Biblical teachings are confirmed in experience and are persuasive because they evoke the consent of reason. At the same time, my own experiencing and reasoning have been so shaped by the religious heritage that nourished me that I can think only as a Christian. Hence, principles from Scripture and from reflection based on experience interact dynamically and unite to form an integrated body of beliefs and value assumptions on which rest all the claims in this essay.[7]

Biblical Principles

1. The Bible does not speak specifically to the issues surrounding physician-assisted death. The problems we face today as a consequence of developments in medical science and technology have created quandaries and dilemmas foreign to the biblical world. Hence, we must search for relevant theological and moral principles in the biblical witness as a whole. In particular, we must look for the highest and best the Bible contains to guide us into this new territory (Philippians 3:8). The love of God for us and the love required of us are basic to Scripture and furnish us with the vital clues we need to deal with the thorniest issues of life and death.

2. A central tenet of the Bible is the goodness of creation (Genesis 1). Life is potentially and essentially good and designed to be

enjoyed. The world offers us treasures of joy and delight that should be savored with enthusiasm and fascination. Dominant in our own deepest experience as well is the intuition that it is good to exist. Every person is made in the image of God and is of immense value. Human existence is rich in meaning and purpose and capable of yielding great pleasure and happiness. This means that life is to be accepted in thanksgiving from the Creator and that we are to seek for ourselves and others the highest possible fulfillment of the potentials for satisfaction and joy given in the good creation. We should do everything in our power to make it possible for every human being to achieve the best and most enjoyable life possible given the unique circumstances, limitations, and abilities of each individual. Consistent with freedom, equality, and justice for all, we should seek the richest, fullest, longest, most meaningful, and happiest life that our resources allow for every person regardless of status or condition.

3. The basic moral principle is that we are to love our neighbors as we love ourselves (Matthew 22:34-40). Love as the chief motive of God's action toward us and of our response to God and of our action in relation to others is at the heart of the New Testament vision (Philippians 2:1-12). To love means to rejoice in the being and to seek the good of the loved one. The well-being of the neighbor is to be regarded as having equal standing with our own as a guide to our motivation and action (Romans 13:8-10). In the presence of suffering, love expresses itself as mercy. Compassion is love's spontaneous response to the torments, terrors, and tribulations of body and mind that mark so much of our existence in this world. We are to be imitators of God, who is rich in mercy and who loves us with a great love (Luke 6:36; Hebrews 2:4, 5:1). The Golden Rule often provides the best guidance about what love and mercy require (Matthew 7:12; Luke 6:31). If we were in a situation of great and hopeless suffering, what would we want others to do for us?

4. While suffering may be the means or the occasion of spiritual growth, our moral duty is to overcome unwanted, involuntary anguish and distress wherever possible and appropriate.[8] We are told that faith enables us to rejoice in our suffering because it builds

character, endurance, and hope (Romans 5:3-5). But we are also told to heal the sick, give sight to the blind, help the lame to walk, and to cast out the demons that afflict us. The healing ministry of Jesus and the imperatives of compassion toward the suffering given to his disciples are fundamental to the Gospels (Matthew 9:35-36, 10:1, 8; Luke 9:1-2).

5. Values are frequently in conflict. The good we seek is often unavoidably accompanied by evil that we wish to avoid but cannot. Sometimes we cannot separate the wheat from the weeds without damaging it (Matthew 13:24-30). Reason and experience confirm what Jesus taught. Moral ambiguity is a pervasive fact of our existence. When it cannot be eluded, we have to seek the best balance of good over evil that the situation permits. Sometimes our choices are such that the best we can do is to avoid the worst evil.

Ethical And Value Judgments

1. What counts is not simply the maintenance of the physical functioning of heart, lungs, and other vital organs in a biological organism but meaningful, purposeful, enjoyable existence as a conscious, thinking, feeling person. It is sometimes justifiable intentionally to end the merely physiological processes of the human body in two circumstances: (a) when the qualities essential to meaningful, purposive personhood — consciousness, thought, self-awareness, emotion, and choice — are forever gone and beyond recovery and (b) when in certain long-term hopeless situations or in a terminal illness life has become an intolerable burden rather than a joyful blessing and no change for the better is possible.

2. Sometimes relief of suffering takes precedence over prolongation of life. Determining when this is the case presents us with some of the most baffling decisions we will ever have to make.

3. Individuals should be given wide latitude in deciding for themselves when death is preferable to a continuing life of misery when relief is impossible. We are also members of society and exist in interdependence with families and communities. Our responsibilities to others must be weighed against our own interests. Nevertheless, when it comes to the point of final decision regarding whether to live or die, the burden of proof is on those who would

take the right of choice away from the sufferer. The state has an interest in protecting the life and liberty of every person and in promoting the best interests of all. In particular, the state should protect individuals against harm, injustice, and abuse at the hands of others. Nevertheless, its laws and actions in promoting these aims should give priority to the rights and liberties of individuals in the ultimate matters pertaining to their own life and death.

The remainder of this essay consists of several parts. First, I present briefly the main arguments for and against physician assistance in dying. After that I offer more extended treatments of the major objections and make the positive case. Finally, I make a proposal as to how we might proceed to legalize assistance in dying in a way that cautiously moves ahead but allows plenty of time for debate and actual experience to instruct us as to whether legalization was wise. Although I touch on a wide variety of issues, the focus is on physician assistance in hastening death for the hopelessly ill. While I take positions that go beyond that, I devote attention primarily to the issues that are at the forefront of current debate.

---

1. The term passive is misleading, since somebody must actually do something to withdraw the life-preserving treatment; for example, either shut off a respirator or remove a feeding tube. Moreover, death is knowingly hastened by this positive activity. Passive euthanasia, however, is a conventional way of speaking that is widely used and is therefore retained here.

2. In some rare and extreme circumstances this could include killing another person, even a stranger, in an emergency situation in which consent cannot be given but in which it would be apparent that the individual would have consented if that had been possible. Here the Golden Rule principle applies. For example, if a person were in great torment in a burning car with no chance whatsoever of survival but could not communicate, it might be moral to kill that person instantly with a gun without explicit consent under the assumption that consent would have been given by the dying person had it been possible.

3. The line between some categories is not always unambiguous or precise. Imagine a terminally-ill patient in great and unrelievable suffering who wants desperately to die. Imagine that a friend offers to kill him. Suppose that the patient, however, respectfully rejects the offer because he or she believes that to

choose death deliberately, no matter what the circumstances, is a grievous sin that would send patient and perpetrator into everlasting punishment. The friend, harboring no such scruples, kills the patient anyway. Can this be regarded as a mercy killing? Was this voluntary or involuntary active euthanasia? One could argue it both ways, since the patient wanted to die but did not wish to be killed. Robert Latimer's killing of his daughter is also hard for me to classify since I do not have all the relevant information.

4. For example, some would permit physician-assisted suicide under carefully controlled and limited conditions but draw the line there and forbid non-physicians to assist others to die in settings that could not be fully regulated. At least, they would not want to legalize these irregular and informal arrangements. Assuming the required physical abilities, of course, persons could be assisted to kill themselves in ways that would be beyond the reach of the justice system.

5. Stephen Hawking, *Black Holes and Baby Universes and Other Essays* (New York: Bantam Books, 1993), 1-26, 157-75.

6. James Rachels, *The End of Life: Euthanasia and Morality* (New York: Oxford University Press, 1986).

7. For a detailed treatment of my theological method and conception of biblical authority, see Kenneth Cauthen, *Toward a New Modernism* (Lanham, Maryland: University Press of America, 1997), vii-xii, 1-75. For a detailed account of my ethical outlook, see Kenneth Cauthen, *Process Ethics: a Constructive System* (Lewiston, New York: Edwin Mellen Press, 1984).

8. I put it in this qualified way because some suffering may be endured or assumed voluntarily. Sometimes suffering may be the necessary and unavoidable means toward good ends that justify the misery involved. Hence, one cannot say that all suffering must be avoided or overcome in every instance, but we generally know when suffering is unavoidable, necessary, and justified and when it is destructive in situations in which it can be overcome. Here, as elsewhere, wisdom is required to sort out all these complexities.

Chapter 3

The Main Arguments: Against And For

Physician-assisted death is a question about which reasonable people equally committed to high ethical principles may sharply disagree. Debate should take place in a context of mutual respect in which the parties to the controversy are willing to admit the limitations of their own views. They should also be open to the truth in the opposing position. It is difficult to formulate a view that contains the truth, the whole truth, and nothing but the truth. I make no such claims for myself but simply set forth the best I know up to now.

In this chapter I present the arguments against and for physician-assisted dying. I have tried to be fair in setting forth the objections to the practice. I have made an effort to put them in the strongest possible form and to give them the full weight they deserve. Those who take a position different from mine make important points that cannot be easily dismissed. In subsequent chapters I will take up in much greater detail some of the main objections and make an extended reply. For the moment it may be useful to present briefly the chief arguments that appear when the subject comes up. I do not claim to have included every idea that has been or could be set forth to oppose or defend physician-assisted dying. Nevertheless, I maintain that the principal points in the debate are to be found here in summary form.

Arguments Against

1. **It violates medical ethics.** The Hippocratic Oath expressly forbids giving deadly medicine to anyone who asks. We should hesitate to give this Oath unquestioned authority, however, since it also requires that physicians swear by Apollo and all the gods and

goddesses. The Oath also forbids the taking of fees for teaching medicine, a precept that is rightly not observed today. This ancient document was written for a past age, but we face circumstances not envisioned long ago. Hence, while it contains much that is of lasting value, it cannot serve for today as an absolute source of authority. Every one of its tenets has to be judged by its merits, and hence mere appeal to it settles nothing.

The American Medical Association has consistently condemned physician-assisted suicide as an unethical practice. Nevertheless, attitudes may be changing. According to recent surveys a majority of doctors in some areas — 60 percent in Oregon, 56 percent in Michigan, and 54 percent in Great Britain — favor the practice in extreme circumstances. According to some studies, between 10 and 15 percent of doctors have assisted patients in committing suicide and at least 2 percent have taken deliberate steps to end the life of patients.[1] A recent article by Dr. David Orentlicher in the prestigious *The New England Journal of Medicine* argued persuasively in favor of physician-assisted suicide.[2] Specialists in law, theology, and ethics are not in agreement on the question.

2. **It undermines trust between doctor and patient.** We expect physicians to heal and preserve life, not to kill on request. I reply that I want to be able to trust my doctor to do what is best for me in every situation. This includes assisting me to die with dignity if life becomes an intolerable burden, and I choose not to live any longer. I would not ask a doctor to do anything illegal, but if physician assistance in dying were permitted by law, I would not want to be abandoned in my final hours by a doctor dedicated to my care.

To put it differently, the trust issue works both ways. It is as probable that doctors might lose the confidence of their patients by an unwillingness to assist them in dying as by their willingness to do so. Physicians establish trust over a period of time by demonstrating themselves to be compassionate, competent, and honest people dedicated to the best interests of their patients and respectful of their wishes. The doctor who has earned trust in this way is not likely to lose it by a willingness to accede to a patient's request for assistance in dying in order to end futile, unendurable suffering.

3. Personal autonomy is not an absolute principle. We do not grant unlimited choice to individuals regarding their own lives. Society makes judgments about practices that are inhumane, dangerous, or of such low moral status that forbidding them is warranted. We wisely do not permit dueling with lethal weapons. We do not allow people to sell themselves into slavery. We require people to wear seat belts and put all sorts of limitations on individuals even when they would be harmed most by their own choices. The conclusion of this line of reasoning is that we should not allow people to choose assistance in dying.

The problem of deciding which areas of life are to be left open to individual choice and which are to be regulated is indeed a difficult one. We have been divided for decades over whether abortion should be prohibited or left to the choice of women with an unwanted pregnancy. Over time social attitudes change about some things. Once dueling was permitted. In the past the government outlawed some sexual acts between consenting adults that were thought to be indecent. We now recognize that this was an indefensible intrusion into the private realm. The question immediately before us is whether individuals should be permitted to choose the time and manner of their deaths in some extreme circumstances.

Let us grant that we are social beings who exist in interdependence with others. Everyone considering a choice to die ought to consider how others would be affected by the decision and to take into account the obligations he or she has to family, friends, and society. We have duties to other people as well as freedom to choose what is best for us. Moreover, we rightly fear the excesses and irrationalities of subjective decision-making by radically empowered individuals. But we should also fear equally or more the power of the government to compel persons unwillingly to endure a wretched existence that in their eyes is worse than death. Hence, in the end, when all factors have been weighed, my claim is that this ultimate decision should be given to the only person who is doing the actual experiencing of a life that has become intolerable and without hope of effective remedy. The burden of proof is on those who would allow the government to deny this choice to those who must live the life and die the death in question.

4. **It is a slippery slope**. In general, this argument maintains that sometimes it is unwise to take a small step, even if it is justified, because it will in principle or in practice lead to other steps that are unacceptable. The **logical** version contends that if we cross the line between withdrawing life-sustaining treatment and even the most restricted forms of assisted suicide, there is no reason in principle not to take other steps that are clearly wrong. If we permit the elderly who are terminally ill and suffering uncontrollably to choose assisted suicide, no logical objection can be raised, for example, against allowing this choice to young people not in danger of dying soon and not in intolerable pain. If we permit assisted suicide, no reason can be given to forbid active euthanasia.

The **empirical** version expresses the fear that, whatever logic might dictate, we are likely to go too far in actual practice. We might eventually be killing off the disabled, the poor, the elderly, abnormal babies, and anyone else who becomes inconvenient. Even if we don't go to that extreme, a process will be set in motion whose momentum could lead to procedures that are obviously unwise and wrong.

Hence, both forms of the slippery-slope argument contend that even if assisted suicide could be justified in a few extreme cases, we must not take that step because it could or would lead to others that are reprehensible. Later on I will deal in considerable detail with the slippery-slope problem. Here I will only make three points briefly.

(a) To say that one should not make a reasonable choice now because it might lead to further moves later is not a sound basis for policy making, unless (1) there is something unavoidable or inevitable about the subsequent steps, and (2) the succeeding moves are clearly wrong. Neither (1) nor (2) is necessarily the case.

(b) The worst fears about the slippery slope are surely groundless given the values that prevail in our society. The guard against slippery-slope disasters is the virtue, character, and good sense of our citizens. On this matter, as on many others, our hope is that reasonable people know when to draw a line between going far enough and going too far.

(c) The fundamental issue is not whether taking one needed and justified step might or will lead to others in the same direction but whether the second and subsequent steps are also needed and justified. This point cannot be overemphasized. It is not self-evident that where the line is now drawn in law and practice (between removing life-support and assisted suicide) is where it should be drawn. Each step has to be considered on its own merits, taking into account all relevant considerations that arise with each new proposal. If it is an error to go too far, it is also an error not to go far enough. The debate is about how far is just right. We should keep our focus on making that determination and not be diverted by dubious claims about slippery slopes.

5. Suicide and killing another person are wrong. Taking a life, whether one's own or another, is a serious matter, and we nearly always regard it as tragic and immensely sad. But are there some instances in which it might be the best thing to do given the extreme circumstances? Many would agree that a captured soldier who possessed valuable military secrets might justifiably commit suicide to avoid revealing them when tortured unmercifully. Nearly everyone recognizes that sometimes it is permissible to cause the death of another. Many, for example, believe that enemy soldiers may be killed in a just war. A majority of people in this country support the death penalty for horrible crimes. Nearly everyone believes that in some situations self-defense justifies killing a would-be murderer. The question, except for absolute pacifists, is whether certain extreme circumstances justify the intentional taking of life. This is exactly the question in relation to providing assistance in dying. The mere fact that assisted dying is suicide or killing does not settle the problem but only poses the issue as to whether deliberately hastening death is morally justified in some circumstances.

6. It violates the crucial difference between passive and active procedures. A decisive moral difference exists between (1) letting nature take its course by ceasing or withholding life-sustaining treatment in hopeless cases and (2) taking active steps that deliberately hasten death. In (1) the cause of death is the underlying fatal disease or condition, while in (2) death is caused by human action. This distinction is examined in great detail later in this essay, but for now I reply that this distinction in and of itself is not morally crucial. To focus here misses a far more important point. The proper question is this: What is the best thing to do under certain extreme circumstances? The answer may be: (1) cease life-sustaining treatment, or (2) do something that will bring about a merciful death that shortens the time of intolerable, unnecessary suffering. The patient may legitimately request either one, and we may morally comply. Death occurs sooner than it otherwise would in either instance as a direct consequence of human choice and agency.

7. **The patient may be depressed temporarily or may undergo a change of mind.** This is a valid concern but not decisive. Depression, when present, should be treated. Patients should be given sufficient time and counseling to make sure their decision represents their enduring wish. At some point, however, we have to decide whether patients are to be permitted to be the authors of their own destiny or not. I readily admit that it is not always easy or simple to determine when patients are competent to make such a momentous decision. I only contend that never allowing dying persons to request assistance in dying is worse and leads to greater abuses than permitting them to do so in certain limited situations.

8. **A misdiagnosis or an unexpected cure could occur.** This is a possibility. Keeping this in mind, however, implies only that we should be extremely cautious, not that we should never act under any circumstances. Moreover, if we always allow for the possibility of an unexpected recovery or a misdiagnosis, it follows that we must do absolutely everything in our power to extend life as long as possible. Hence, we would never withdraw life-sustaining treatment even though the case looked totally hopeless if so doing hastened death ever so slightly. For everyone who will not go that far, the problem is to determine exactly what circumstances define a situation that is truly beyond human remedy and hence make it morally permissible either to cease treatment or to hasten death.

9. **Bad consequences would follow.** Guidelines would inevitably be transgressed. Mistakes would be made. If they had the option of choosing to die, patients might feel guilty for staying alive and continuing to be a financial and emotional burden on their families. They might feel their lives had little value if society had provided a way to kill them. Families might be tempted to approve administered death for their terminally-ill members out of exhaustion and financial stress or even out of less worthy motives such as greed or hostility. Doctors might be tempted to consent to the easier way of administering lethal medicine instead of providing compassionate care under extreme conditions. We might all become more callous about death and less committed to the care of the terminally ill once we got used to the idea of assisted death as a solution for life's miseries. The option of deliberately hastening death might lessen efforts to provide maximum pain relief and comfort for the dying. Poor people and minorities would be particularly vulnerable to the temptation for society to urge the death solution as a cheaper alternative to providing better care.

These are valid concerns, and no system can avoid all abuse. But all the pressures that might be felt by patients or urged on them by families or institutions already exist with regard to the approved practice of withdrawing life-sustaining treatment. The poor may be especially vulnerable to such influences. Moreover, because doctors can give large doses of painkillers that also hasten death, the present system already allows for covert instances of assisted death. Leaving aside flagrant violations of acceptable practice that are never discovered, abuses are possible in the murky areas left up to private decisions where one effect — hastened death — can be justified by the other effect — relief of pain. Fewer abuses would occur if all these areas were open to scrutiny and regulation. Far from lessening efforts to manage the suffering of the dying, the option of assisted death might well inspire greater efforts to make patients comfortable, so that they would not be driven to the extreme of wanting to die. The main abuse, however, is that by denying terminally-ill patients a choice to die in hopeless situations, we consign those whose suffering cannot be relieved to needless, pointless agony.

10. **It is God's place to decide the time and place of death.** I reply that assistance in dying is a moral issue that has to be resolved on the basis of principles we use to deal with every other question about right and wrong, not a special case. Nearly everyone agrees that sometimes it is legitimate to take the life of another and thus determine the time and place of that person's death. No special principle exempts assisted suicide or active euthanasia from other circumstances in which we have to determine when taking the life of another is justified and when it is not.

Moreover, the implication is not only that we should never deliberately hasten death, but also that we should never interfere with the course of any life-threatening condition. If a person is bleeding to death from an accidental cut, should we not just watch and let death occur? To intervene would challenge God's prerogative to determine the time and place of death. If someone objects that we are obligated to preserve life but never to take it, that shifts the argument away from the original claim and merely identifies the issue that is in dispute.

Sometimes it is said that deliberately causing a patient's death is "playing God." It is incumbent on anyone who makes this argument to spell out the principles that tell us when we have assumed a prerogative reserved for God. If this claim is based on intuition or feeling, as it often seems to be, it is not decisive, since others have different intuitions and feelings. When the phrase is given content, it usually involves a commendable warning against pride based on the finitude and fallibility of human beings. Less convincingly, it may indicate a list of areas that we should not pry into or interfere with, such as the beginning or end of life or the fundamental secrets of life itself.[3] At best, "playing God" identifies a point of reference around which discussion may take place. At worst, when one person accuses another of transgressing the boundary between divine and human spheres of action, it means nothing more than that the latter is willing to go further in intervening in life processes than the former. In any case, "playing God" is not a self-evident, self-defining premise that settles questions merely by being invoked.

11. **Hastening death to escape suffering denies the role that suffering plays in God's plan.** An extreme view that every instance of suffering is divinely intended or purposeful would not only rule out assisted death but would also forbid efforts to alleviate any suffering. It is true that affliction can and often does serve a moral or spiritual purpose. Many have testified that suffering led them to greater maturity and a deeper relation with God and others. It is not a contradiction, however, to believe also that we have an obligation to ease pain and misery to the fullest degree our knowledge and skill permit. Exceptions to this rule may occur if the suffering in question is assumed voluntarily for some good reason or is a necessary and justified means to some desired end. Even some who insist that in God's purpose suffering plays a necessary and divinely-intended role in developing us as moral beings also contend that it is our duty to reduce or eliminate it wherever possible. In fact, one way that suffering serves its divinely-intended function in this view is that it inspires us to acts of mercy in overcoming the afflictions of our neighbors.[4] Hence, whatever we may reasonably believe about the positive role that suffering can play and is divinely intended to play in life does not mean that we are interfering with God's intention when we seek to diminish the unwanted and unnecessary torments and agonies of this earthly life. If this is true, it is legitimate to raise the question as to whether in certain extreme, hopeless circumstances relieving suffering by hastening death is permissible. I maintain that it is.[5]

Arguments For

Deciding what is right is especially difficult when the permissibility of deliberately ending a human life is involved. In these drastic situations the normal rules of morality are stretched to the breaking point. Self-defense against a would-be murderer, killing enemy soldiers in a just war, capital punishment for the most horrendous crimes, intentional suicide by a spy to prevent torture or a coerced confession of vital military information, killing a berserk man who is systematically murdering a line of hostages — all these instances pose questions that severely test our moral wisdom.

Nearly everyone would agree that in some of the cases listed it would be legitimate to end a life deliberately. This fact tells us that suicide and killing are not always and necessarily regarded as wrong. It depends upon the circumstances. Now enters the question of physician assistance in dying. I argue that under some carefully defined situations it is morally permissible for a physician to assist a person in hastening death to end unwanted, intolerable, unnecessary suffering.

1. In some circumstances individual autonomy takes precedence over the interest of the state in protecting life. The strongest case for allowing patients to choose death over the continuation of life can be made when they are terminally ill and are undergoing intolerable suffering that cannot be controlled. A strong case can also be made for competent people not terminally ill whose lives have become permanently unbearable without remedy. The possibility of choosing to die would be available in both cases only as a last resort when all appropriate efforts to make life worth living have been exhausted.

Suppose a person in either situation says, "My life has ceased to be worth living. I cannot stand it any longer. I want to end it now to avoid further pain, indignity, torment, and despair." We would want to urge consultation with physicians, clergy, lawyers, therapists, family, and others so that such a serious and irreversible decision could be made after sufficient time has passed and every alternative thoroughly weighed. In the end, however, after all alternatives have been thoroughly considered, we should give primacy to the right of suffering people to decide when life has become an unendurable hardship. It is they and no one else who are undergoing the actual torment.

To whom, if not the subject of the suffering, should be given this awesome power? Who is more qualified than I and who has more right than I to decide whether to live or die, since it is I who live my life and die my death? The burden of proof rests on the claim that this prerogative should be overridden by obligations to family and society. Above all, the burden rests upon the state to justify its right to overrule the choice of individuals and to force an unwanted existence upon tormented souls.

Persons permanently suffering intolerably did not choose to be in this state. Moreover, nothing they or anyone else can do will make life bearable. In some cases they may have acted foolishly in ways that led to their grievous condition, but they did not deliberately choose the condition itself. When death becomes preferable to life under circumstances that cannot be changed, individuals should be able to avail themselves of the only remedy for their unendurable existence that is available. When any reasonable possibility of meaningful, enjoyable existence lies ahead, the desire will be for life. Therefore, every possible effort must be made to make continuing life preferable to death. Obviously, people who are mentally ill or severely depressed present special cases. We must proceed with utmost caution when we are dealing with people who are not near death without closing the door entirely. In the end, however, the burden of proof rests on those who would deny individuals the right to make the ultimate decisions about their own living and dying.

These are difficult questions, I grant. Moreover, as I have urged repeatedly, we must do everything possible to make life preferable to death. In particular, patients should have their pain and other types of physical and emotional agony relieved to the fullest extent that modern medical knowledge and skill permit. Moreover, they should be surrounded by caring people who provide love, understanding, and assistance in making life endurable and rewarding. We must make sure any choice to die is a persisting one on the part of a fully-informed, competent person after thorough consideration of all options, taking everything into account. But in the end I see no reason to deny individuals the right to make that final decision. In particular, I find no justification for allowing the government to forbid that choice. The appropriate role of the state is to institute proper procedures and safeguards to prevent mistakes and abuses, not to forbid the choice to die when the requisite conditions are met.

2. **The role of the physician is to do what is best for the patient in every situation, and that may include hastening death in some extreme circumstance upon the voluntary request of the dying.** Many argue that doctors are committed to preserving

and enhancing life, not ending it deliberately. To assist a patient in hastening death would violate the deepest obligations and values of the medical profession. If one defines the role of the physician solely in terms of healing and preserving life and limits it strictly to that, assisting a patient to die obviously violates the job description. That, however, is the wrong way to go about defining the scope of the physician's responsibility.

The proper question is this: What is the best thing doctors can do to help their patients in whatever circumstances arise, given their special knowledge and skills? In nearly every case the answer will be to heal, to prolong life, to reduce suffering, to restore health and physical well-being, i.e., to preserve and enhance life. But in some extreme, hopeless circumstances, the best service a physician can render may be, upon request, to hasten death by deliberate means in order to relieve intolerable, unnecessary suffering that makes life unbearable as judged by the patient. This would be an enlargement of the physician's role, not a contradiction of it.

3. **Sometimes ending suffering by hastening death takes precedence over extending life.** Providing assistance in dying is so troubling because it involves an agonizing conflict between values. Life is a wonderful gift full of the promise of pleasure, joy, happiness, and love. But circumstances may turn life into a heartbreaking, hopeless burden filled with suffering, pain, and despair. We desire to live, but in some situations death may be preferable to the continuation of an intolerable existence. If some person comes to that dreadful conclusion, what is our duty? The moral imperative forbids us to kill, but it also enjoins us to be merciful. While insisting that we must make every effort possible to guard against abuse, I sorrowfully conclude that, at a patient's request, it may sometimes be more merciful and loving to end suffering than to extend a joyless, unendurable life. Circumstances arise in which it is in no one's interest to prolong the existence of someone whose potential for desirable life has been thoroughly exhausted beyond recovery.

4. **When death becomes preferable to life, everyone would benefit if it were legal to show mercy.** Compassion and benevolence demand that we legalize assisted death for the sake of the

afflicted and those who love them. The most powerful argument in favor of physician-assisted death comes from the families of those who have witnessed loved ones die in extreme agony. When medical science has done all it can and death has not yet brought merciful relief, family members suffer a sense of powerlessness and despair as they watch in horror someone they love dearly writhe in excruciating pain as they all wait and hope for a quick end to his or her torment. That these extreme cases are rare is indeed fortunate, but it does not render less important the appalling plight of those who must live — hopelessly and helplessly — through such distress. Both the patient and the patient's family and friends are unnecessarily put in an awful position. By legalizing assisted death, we show mercy to the patient and provide a great benefit to family and friends. Everyone is better off.

The most forlorn of all are those who agonize over whether to take action in violation of the law to end the life of someone dear to them who pleads and prays for death. A few in desperation, unable to stand it any longer, take a gun or a pillow and do what they dread and hate to do but must do. They are driven to act in order to bring relief to a parent or child or spouse who is glad for the intervention but is fearful of the legal consequences for those who have shown them mercy. Not every mercy killing can be justified. Some cases are so complex and involve such an intertwining of conflicting values that we find ourselves on a knife edge between approving and disapproving. Nevertheless, compassion for those who show mercy will deter us from making absolute judgments while recognizing how dangerous it is for one person to take the life of another. At the same time we can sympathize with the tragic and ambiguous circumstances in which people find themselves being torn between showing mercy and killing.

You have seen them, heard them, or read about them. Their faces are sometimes hidden and their voices disguised as they tell their sad stories. They must witness carefully to what has happened because the law condemns their compassion and calls them murderers. Yet they loved the deceased with all their hearts and were moved to do the dreadful deed out of pure benevolence. Sue Rodriguez found a way to get help in dying, but she had to do it in a way that would not implicate those who assisted her in a crime. Austin Bastable wanted a legal way to end his suffering but had to resort to the notorious Dr. Jack Kevorkian when no other options were available to him. Robert Latimer said that he killed his twelve-year-old daughter who had been afflicted from birth with cerebral palsy as an "act of mercy" to save her from a life of constant pain and misery. Our hearts are torn apart trying to decide whether his dreadful deed was justified by mercy or whether he committed murder.

Even as final revisions were being made to this book, another tragic instance came to light. On February 20, 1998, John Bement was convicted of manslaughter by a Buffalo, New York, court for feeding poisonous pudding to his wife. He faces a possible sentence of up to fifteen years in prison. Judith Bement suffered from ALS (Lou Gehrig's disease) and her body wasted away until she was completely paralyzed. Finally, she reached a point that she could stand it no longer. Family and friends reported that she had begged for assistance in committing suicide "hundreds of times." Mr. Bement resisted for a long time, insisting that she would get better. Finally, he gave in and did what his wife pleaded for him to do. As a result a split has occurred between two daughters who have taken opposing positions on the matter. I fail to see how legalizing assisted suicide could produce worse consequences than the situation we have now, as this case and many others like it so vividly demonstrate.[6]

Physicians are more fortunate in that they can take refuge in the principle of the "double effect" and write on the death certificate the cause of death. Many of us have heard doctors report that they have, out of compassion and mercy, given heavy doses of morphine to relieve the pain of patients who were near to an inevitable death. They knew full well that what they did would hasten the end. This is currently permitted, since the primary aim is, it is said, to relieve pain and not to kill. But it would not be right, we are told, to do the very same thing with the primary aim of hastening death. I do not accept this reasoning.

Why do we force good people full of love, mercy, and compassion to such extreme measures to bring an end to hopeless suffering when no cure or relief is possible for the dearest people on earth to them? Why do we force physicians to justify their mercy in hastening death by denying that they did it for that reason, when we all know what is really going on? I am a theologian, a philosopher, an ethicist, and a Baptist minister. I hold our moral, legal, and theological heritage in high regard. But there are times when we need to rethink received wisdom by subjecting our principles, codes, and traditions to a fresh exposure to real-life experience. Sometimes ideals that are designed to protect and enhance life may actually degrade life and be the source of unnecessary suffering. So it is, I believe, with the prohibition of physician-assisted death under any and all circumstances. We can provide an opportunity for patients in certain extreme and rare cases under strictly regulated conditions to manage their dying without endangering our reverence for life. In so doing we can provide a way to be merciful to the dying without branding those who show mercy as criminals. We can avoid the agony of family members and of physicians who must do in secret what love and compassion urge upon them and thus serve the dying while honoring the living.

In the next three chapters I will deal in more detail with the most formidable arguments against physician-assisted death and show that they are not sound. I will begin with what is usually called the slippery-slope objection.

---

1. Ezekiel Emanuel, "Euthanasia and Assisted Suicide," *Harvard Risk Management Foundation* (May 1995).

2. David Orentlicher, "The Legalization of Physician-Assisted Suicide," *The New England Journal of Medicine* (August 29, 1996).

3. See *Cloning Human Beings*, Report of the National Bioethics Advisory Committee (June 1997), 44-5.

4. An impressive statement of the view that God has created the world to be a laboratory of soul-making in which suffering plays an essential role can be

found in John Hick, *Evil and the God of Love* (San Francisco: Harper & Row, 1978).

5. The role of suffering in human life is far too complex to be treated fully here. I have dealt in detail with the subject in *The Many Faces of Evil: Reflections on the Sinful, the Tragic, the Demonic, and the Ambiguous* (Lima, Ohio: CSS Publishing Co., 1997).

6. *Democrat and Chronicle*, Rochester, New York (March 9, 1998), 5B.

Chapter 4

The Slippery-Slope Argument: The Logical Version

One of the most powerful objections to assisted death is the danger posed by the slippery slope. Nearly everyone worries about this. Three reasons can be given to justify an extended treatment to untangle the issues. (1) Opponents of assisted death make a great deal of the slippery-slope argument. (2) The slippery-slope argument raises important questions about the extent to which individual self-determination takes precedence over the interest of the government in protecting life. (3) Since I go further than the initial steps I concentrate on, I need to defend myself against the charge that my own position demonstrates the danger of the slippery slope.

This argument comes in two varieties: the logical and the empirical. Both types of slippery-slope arguments are subtle and complex. Hence, I devote two chapters to the slippery-slope objection to assisted death in order that the scope and limits of its validity may be determined.

The Logical Version

The logical form claims that the endorsement of a certain practice entails that other related practices become reasonable. Since the more extensive applications are obviously wrong, the first action must not be taken. The typical argument for providing assistance in dying initially assumes a narrow scope of application that presupposes four conditions: (1) the patient is near death, (2) in unbearable, unmanageable pain or suffering, (3) mentally competent to make a voluntary request, and (4) the choice of death endures after thorough reflection. Some opponents are willing to admit that in a few instances in which these restricted conditions are met, physician-assisted suicide is warranted. However, they maintain that we must not take the step of legalizing the practice because its application cannot logically be limited to the stated criteria.

My reply will revolve around two claims. First of all, wider extensions are not necessarily or inevitably implied. Just because a practice can be warranted by a given set of principles in one set of circumstances does not always mean that related but different practices can be authorized by those same principles. Additional or dissimilar considerations may have to be taken into account when other practices are examined that may lead to a different conclusion. Each new issue has to be judged on its own merits in terms of all the distinctive factors involved.

In the second place, even if wider extensions beyond the restricted case are sometimes logically implied, we still have to decide whether they are justified. We have to distinguish between the logical implications of arguments and their moral soundness. They are not the same thing. This is the essential point that I will repeatedly make since it is so crucial. The slippery-slope argument assumes that some or all of the moves beyond the first are obviously or demonstrably wrong and therefore must be forbidden. But this is exactly what the debate is about and cannot simply be assumed in advance. An argument for some restricted practice may imply wider applications that are as ethically valid as the original application.

In order to prove their point, those who suspect a slippery slope must find an explicit or implicit axiom in a proposal that has implications beyond the original case. A premise must be present that when spelled out extends the initial application. It is here that the logical version of slippery-slope arguments gets slippery. If one maintained, for example, that the tacit principle in assisted dying, even on the narrow grounds stated, is the legitimizing of the taking of innocent life, then obviously this would open the door as wide as the most extravagant critics claim. However, while the taking of innocent life is involved in the situation, to abstract that component and make broad deductions from it ignores the whole set of conditions that have been previously specified as justifying the taking of innocent life. To say that it is sometimes acceptable to take innocent life does not mean that it is always right to do so.

We readily see the fallacy of this type of ambitious slippery-slope argument in other situations that are more familiar. Most people recognize that taking the life of a violent aggressor to preserve one's own life is permissible if this is the only way to keep from being murdered. Yet no reasonable person argues that this is a slippery slope that logically entails the proposition that one can kill the driver who pulls into a parking place ahead of you. Yet implicit in self-defense at some level of abstraction is the principle that one citizen may kill another. This principle, without qualification, would include killing someone who took the one remaining parking place that you had your heart set on. We rightly recognize that there are relevant moral differences between self-defense against a would-be murderer and killing a person who steals a parking place.

The restricted argument for physician-assisted dying does not logically authorize the killing of all innocent people but only those who meet all requirements stipulated. It is illegitimate to abstract some remote generalized feature and make deductions from it as if all the other factors don't matter. They do matter. Circumstances alter cases. Hence, each situation must be taken up on its own with all its necessary features intact. Each situation has a configuration of components that are essential to it, all of which must be honored. To show that a slippery slope is present, it would be necessary to show that no relevant moral differences exist between a first step that is justified and subsequent steps that are not. If no relevant differences arise, the subsequent steps should also be acceptable. If relevant differences are present, they must be taken into account to determine whether they make it necessary to draw a line that should not be crossed.

A more formidable version of the slippery-slope argument contends that the more general postulate in the defense of assisted dying is the principle of individual autonomy. If one believes that an individual has an unlimited right to determine when life has become intolerable, then obviously this cannot logically be restricted to cases in which the patient is dying and in intractable physical pain or untreatable misery. People in all sorts of conditions might conclude that life had become hopelessly intolerable and opt for death. Young people, for example, with an incurable progressing degenerative disease with many years of unendurable existence ahead might decide at some point to die rather than go on. Here the slippery-slope objection is stronger. Nevertheless, this expansive view of personal autonomy is not logically essential to the original argument. One could argue that only when the conditions of competence, imminent demise, and intractable suffering exist does the patient have the right to choose death. It all depends on how much weight is given to individual autonomy in relation to other principles in one case as compared to others.

We can imagine a situation in which the slippery-slope argument has validity. If the principle of individual autonomy is assumed to be absolute, the sole consideration, limited by no other principle, then obviously death can be chosen by anyone who merely makes that choice for whatever reasons are convincing to that individual. Hence, if that principle is a hidden but operative assumption when the limited case is made for dying patients in intolerable misery, then a slippery slope is truly present. If, however, one maintains that the right to choose life or death for oneself is an important value but not the only one that has to be taken into account, a different situation emerges. One then has to ask what these other values, rights, and principles are and how they are to be weighed against individual autonomy. Many factors enter into the determination of what is morally licit. Each situation has to be judged on the basis of the principles, facts, and circumstances that are relevant to it. An argument to limit the right to choose assistance in hastening death to certain extreme instances is logically secure against slippery-slope arguments if that argument specifies the mandatory principles that come into play when the issue of assisted death arises under various circumstances. The argument may or may not be valid or convincing, but it is not subject to slippery-slope objections.

Illustrating the issues surrounding the slippery slope in this respect is the argument of Yale Kamisar. He maintains that once assisted suicide has been established, even in its most restricted form, no principled reason can be given for not extending it far beyond that into clearly unacceptable applications. Underlying this line of reasoning is that "the basic argument for assisted suicide is 'personal autonomy' or 'self-determination.' "[1] If the right to a doctor's aid is granted to the terminally ill, he asks why the same right should not be granted to those who are undergoing great suffering but not terminally ill. If we permit doctors to provide the means for patients to kill themselves (physician-assisted suicide), he asks why we should not permit them to go ahead and administer a lethal injection (voluntary active euthanasia). In each case, he answers that if we take the first step, the other steps logically follow. If the underlying principle is the right of individuals to choose their own destiny, no principled reason can be given for not allowing them to choose death for whatever reasons that for them make life unbearable. Hence, Kamisar rejects assisted suicide even in its most limited form, since the logic of the principle of self-determination leads to an unlimited right of persons to have other people kill them upon their request.

Framed in this way, he is correct. That is exactly the point I have been making. However, I have also urged that one might reasonably argue that other factors limit the scope of self-determination. In this connection let us note that Professor Kamisar agrees that the terminally ill have a right to demand the withdrawal of life-sustaining equipment, even though they will die sooner. Does this not put him on a slippery slope, so that no principled argument can be given for not extending that right to include requesting assistance in dying? His implied answer is no. Kamisar argues that one can draw a line between the two and offers a number of reasons to justify the one but not the other. He argues that the circumstances are morally and medically different in the two cases. Hence, patient refusal of life-sustaining procedures must be honored, but the request for medicines that the patient can use to commit suicide can be legitimately denied.

Notice, however, that the logic of his reasoning is that personal autonomy is an important principle, but it can be limited by circumstances and contexts. That is the exact line of reasoning I have followed to argue that granting the right to assisted death under very limited circumstances does not necessarily create a slippery slope that leads to the unrestricted right to persons to have others kill them. The formal nature of his reasoning is identical to mine. We still need to examine the material content of his reasoning to determine whether the difference he finds between withdrawing life support and assisted suicide can withstand rigorous scrutiny. I claim that it cannot. But his own line of thought shows that slippery slopes are not inevitable. One can reasonably draw lines at various points depending on the relevant factors that exist in different sets of circumstances and the weight assigned to them. The question always is: Where must we draw the line? It is not apparent to me that where Kamisar draws the line is the appropriate place.

The way slippery-slope arguments go depends a great deal on how we set them up. If someone argues against instituting a warranted practice because it would logically lead to unwarranted practices, it is easy to create another situation and use it to show that something the opponent favors is also susceptible to slippery-slope logic. Let us imagine another starting point. Suppose we begin with the principle that we must do absolutely everything possible right down to the last moment to keep a dying patient alive as long as is humanly possible, sparing no expense. If that were the rule in effect, would Kamisar argue against modifying that position ever so slightly because it might lead to the slippery slope he fears that would eventually permit all sorts of unwarranted practices? No, he would not. Kamisar gives good, convincing reasons why patients should be permitted to demand withdrawal of life-sustaining treatment in hopeless cases, resulting in a quicker death. But he insists that the line be drawn there.

Thus, he would deny a dying patient in great unrelievable agony the right to request the assistance of a physician in committing suicide. Why? If a patient has a right to order the cessation of life-sustaining procedures even though it results in a quicker death, on what principle should we deny the extension of that freedom of choice to include a request for deliberate means to hasten death? If personal autonomy applies in the first instance, why should it not apply in the second? Kamisar thinks that relevant differences pertain between them that permit choice in the one but not in the other. Whether the reasons he gives are valid is not the issue here. The point at the moment is that we do not necessarily draw lines on the basis of one principle alone but on all the pertinent factors that arise in a particular situation. Kamisar and I agree on that point. Furthermore, Kamisar even admits that, in a few cases, it might be legitimate to permit physician-assisted suicide to dying patients. But he defines himself as a rule utilitarian who believes that better consequences will follow if we make a rule against assisted suicide in all cases, rather than, as an act utilitarian, make a judgment for or against it in each particular case.[2] I find his reasoning here strange and utterly unconvincing. First of all, I think that in general the contest between rule ethics and act ethics is a standoff with no clear victor. Many general rules require exceptions, and a general rule is implicit in every decision made about a particular act.[3] Beyond that, I suggest that we make a different rule. Instead of a rule that forbids assisted suicide in all cases, why not formulate a rule that forbids assisted suicide in all cases except those that meet the conditions that Kamisar actually thinks would warrant it. But for Kamisar to accept that rule would create a dilemma, since it would by his reasoning set us on a slippery slope. Yet not to accept the rule requires Kamisar to deny assisted suicide to those he thinks actually deserve it.

In short, I conclude that no slippery slope is necessarily logically present in the initial case that restricts physician-assisted dying to mentally competent, fully informed patients whose death is imminent, who suffer intolerably from misery that cannot be relieved, and whose voluntary request endures after thorough rational consideration. If one insists that (1) all these requirements are essential to the legitimizing of physician-assisted death in every instance and that (2) relevant moral differences obtain between the restricted situation and subsequent steps, then no principle of logic necessitates its extension. We all draw lines somewhere. Wider implications may arise in particular cases depending on the assumptions actually underlying the arguments of a given advocate. In short, it all depends on the postulates that are actually present, not those arbitrarily imposed or wildly imagined to be necessarily presupposed.

To put it differently, imagine two proponents of assisted suicide. One makes argument A, and the other makes argument B.

Argument A: The principle of individual autonomy gives a terminally-ill patient the right to choose physician-assisted suicide when and only when the following four conditions apply: (1) The patient is near death and beyond hope. (2) The patient is competent and makes a voluntary choice. (3) The patient is undergoing intolerable suffering that cannot be alleviated. (4) The choice is an enduring one after being fully informed and giving the matter thorough consideration.

Argument B: The principle of individual autonomy gives a person the unlimited right to choose physician-assisted suicide under any and all circumstances in which he or she determines that life has become unbearable. Therefore, it follows that, of course, a terminally-ill patient has the right to choose assisted suicide when the four conditions specified in A are present.

Personally, I believe that A is too restricted and that the initial premise in B goes too far, although I am closer to B than to A. Here, however, we are dealing only with the logical implications of each contention. I maintain that argument A involves no slippery-slope. Argument B is more complicated. If someone makes the case initially for physician-assisted suicide only when the four conditions in A apply, but the underlying principle is unlimited personal autonomy, then obviously no principled reason can be given for not extending that right to others than the terminally ill. The reason is simple. The initial premise in B explicitly states that anyone who prefers to die, for whatever reasons, has the right to physician-assisted suicide. Strictly speaking, however, a slippery slope is involved only if the initial premise in B is operative but unacknowledged or not stated. If the initial premise is explicitly acknowledged, then those who hold it are simply contending that physician-assisted death is permissible in a wide variety of cases including but not limited to the restricted case assumed in A. That view has to be dealt with on its own terms. The assertion in B of an unlimited extension of the right of personal autonomy may not be morally sound, since it gives so much weight to that principle in relation to other relevant considerations. It involves no slippery slope, however, if the full implications are stated from the outset. Hence, the slippery-slope objection may but does not necessarily apply in a given case. It all depends on how the argument is framed.

To conclude, one point of utmost importance has to be made once more. **The fundamental issue is not whether taking one step logically leads to other steps but whether the next steps are justified by valid value premises and factual considerations.** Kamisar and others assume that physician-assisted death is highly questionable and nearly always forbidden even when the four conditions in A are present and that any wider applications are obviously wrong. That is what the crucial debate is all about in the last analysis, not about slippery slopes that may or may not be present.

Have I despite myself actually illustrated in my own thinking the reality and the dangers of the slippery slope? After all, I not only argue for physician-assisted suicide but also make a case for physician-administered death. Furthermore, I would make it available not only to the terminally ill whose suffering cannot be controlled but also to some persons not terminally ill for whom life has become permanently and often increasingly intolerable. I deny that a slippery slope is involved here. I do not begin with a small step and then find myself logically forced to take additional steps beyond that contrary to my original intentions. Rather, I begin by laying out the principles that I take to be compelling and simply indicate what they imply for a variety of circumstances. I believe the case for assisted death is stronger in some cases than others, but I do not begin with a restricted application and then find myself obliged by logic to go further than I had intended on the basis of the initial premises. I lay out all the implications from the outset. No hidden or unacknowledged premises are present that, when exposed, lead me inevitably beyond the first case I argue for. I am not forced by the necessities of correct thinking to accept wider applications that I had first rejected. I make everything I defend explicit from the beginning. While others may reasonably disagree with my position on any and all issues, they cannot accuse me of putting myself on a slippery slope.

I do argue that it is possible for others to make a case for physician-assisted suicide for the terminally ill only that is not susceptible to slippery-slope logic if they state their position carefully from the beginning. Finally, I do admit that some who make the restricted case for physician-assisted suicide may put themselves on a slippery slope if they actually operate with implicit assumptions that they do not originally acknowledge or may not even be aware of at first. In this case, those who argue for the restricted case only may find themselves forced to admit that logic compels them to go further than they had intended into positions they resist. It is against this group only that the slippery-slope objection applies.

The next chapter will examine in detail the empirical version of the slippery-slope argument. Then I will add some final reflections about the slippery-slope problem in general.

---

1. Yale Kamisar, "Against Assisted Suicide — Even in a Very Limited Form," Testimony to the Committee on the Judiciary, United States House of Representatives, April 29, 1996.

2. Rule ethics contends that we can derive general rules that are valid for every occasion. Act ethics contends that since moral choices have to be made under so many different circumstances, it is better not to make binding general rules but to decide what is right in every particular case. A utilitarian believes that rightness is determined by which consequences will achieve the greatest good. See my *Process Ethics: A Constructive System* (Lewiston, New York: Edwin Mellen Press, 1984), 77-82, for more detail. See also, William K. Frankena, *Ethics*, 2nd ed. (Englewood Cliffs, New Jersey: Prentice-Hall, 1973), 23-7, 35-43.

3. For example, "killing is wrong" is a general rule. But most people recognize that it requires exceptions, for example, in certain cases of self-defense or in war. If we start within a particular instance in which we conclude that the moral imperative forbids us to kill, that implies the general rule that killing is wrong.

Chapter 5

The Slippery-Slope Argument: The Empirical Version

The logical form of the slippery-slope argument deals with the implications of principles of thought. It has to do with the realm of theory and the rules of sound and consistent thinking. The empirical version of the slippery-slope argument moves into the realm of practice and voices fears about what will or might happen in real life if physician-assisted suicide were to be permitted even in a limited form. While we must be on guard against the dangers involved in legalizing assisted death, I maintain that the slippery-slope argument in this form is no more convincing than the logical version.

The Empirical Version

While some objectors might admit that slippery slopes are not always logically inescapable, they contend that as a matter of fact, once the first step is taken, other steps will or might be taken, and this would be disastrous. Some are afraid that assisted suicide voluntarily chosen by the dying presses inexorably toward the dreadful possibility that death might be deliberately administered to all sorts of people who will have little choice in the matter. They are especially concerned about vulnerable members of society such as the poor, minorities, the disabled, and the elderly, who might be killed for the convenience of society or family members. In its extreme form this objection has little merit. Unless the values of our society change drastically, that outcome is not a probability we need to worry about.

The troubling concern is not that anyone would ever explicitly propose the intentional killing of the elderly, the disabled, the poor, or any other group of innocent, defenseless people against their will. It is rather that once assisted death, no matter how restricted, is legalized, subtle pressures might arise to extend its application. For example, the power of money could come into play. Insurance companies, HMOs, hospitals, nursing homes, and others who stand to gain by reducing the cost of caring for the seriously ill might seek ways to put delicate or disguised pressure on the dying or their families to choose death sooner rather than later in the name of "quality of life." As abhorrent as this sounds, we must be realistically alert to the possibility of exploitation and initiate the most stringent safeguards possible to prevent it. It is possible, of course, that other abuses could be instigated by scheming or exhausted family members, physicians, and health care institutions for a variety of monetary and non-monetary reasons.

Obviously, we should fear pressures on patients to choose death from those who stand to gain by that choice. The fact is, however, that these same dangers exist already with regard to expensive treatments that might prolong life. Patients have the right to refuse or withdraw treatment, even if it shortens life. Therefore, we should worry now about pressures that might persuade patients to order the removal of life-support systems or to decline other treatments that would cost somebody a lot of money. Abuses can occur under any set of conditions. No policy or set of laws can be guaranteed in advance to be foolproof. Vigilance is essential to keep mistreatment to an absolute minimum. Moreover, opponents who warn us of the dangers of permitting a right to choose death in the absence of guaranteed health care must be listened to. The proper response, however, is not to deny the former but to establish the latter as well.

The strongest feature of the empirical argument perhaps is that once we have legitimized the taking of innocent life in any circumstance whatsoever, a gradual process will or might take place in which we become more callous about human life. A hardening of attitudes could occur once we get used to the idea of deliberately putting an end to someone's life. While initially we might restrict voluntary active euthanasia to those who are suffering greatly, in time it would not seem so bad to kill others whose situation was not so desperate if they request it.

The empirical version of the slippery-slope argument is unprovable, impossible to disprove, and difficult to assess. When new ground is being explored, we cannot be certain what the ultimate consequences will be. Nevertheless, while analogies may be deceptive, they may be helpful if well chosen. Most states threaten capital punishment for the most brutal crimes. Does anyone fear that this is a slippery slope that will eventually have the state killing its citizens for a parking violation? Does the fact that people may voluntarily donate bodily organs upon their death set in motion an inevitable process that leads to the involuntary harvesting of hearts and livers from the poor and the disabled who are still living? Once the practice of granting a state license is established for anything, for example, to practice medicine or drive a car on public highways, surely this is a slippery slope that will inevitably lead to the requirement of a license for six-year-old children to ride a tricycle inside their homes. Surely we must not regulate the most repugnant forms of pornography that feature the rape and dismemberment of children and the violent degradation of women, because, alas, the end result would be the total abolition of free speech.

Most of us do not fear these absurd extremes. The reason is that we have confidence that our citizens have the virtue and the intelligence in the long run to avoid them. If they are fully informed and think it through, decent people will stop short of excesses that lack grounding in either reason or morality. Our hope with respect to assisted death as well is that sensible people can make sound judgments that recognize the crucial differences between what is acceptable and what is clearly not. We have a set of basic values inherited from our past to guide us in making these judgments. Society is constantly rethinking its traditions to discover what is more just, more compassionate, and more desirable. This is going on now with respect to physician assistance in dying.

Let us grant that it is not always easy to know where to draw the line. Sometimes situations are ambiguous, so that every choice involves a mixture of good and bad. Moreover, equally wise people may disagree vigorously about moral issues. Our society is deeply torn now over abortion, affirmative action, prayer in schools, and many other problems. Nevertheless, surely we can count on the basic good sense and moral sensibilities of the majority of people to avoid the extremes that offend our basic sensibilities. If we cannot, then no one is secure from outrage anyway with respect to assistance in dying and many other questions as well. The quality of our common life is always dependent on the rectitude and discernment of citizens to know when we have moved from the reasonable and defensible into the realm of the irresponsible and the heartless.

It is bad policy to refuse to take a prudent and needed step now because of some extreme that might possibly come about at some time in the future. The cost of not legalizing assisted dying under restricted, carefully safeguarded conditions is to consign some hopelessly ill patients — fortunately not very many — to needless suffering because of greatly exaggerated if not groundless fears. The abuses now actually occurring call for a remedy that will allow mercy to do its work in the open rather than secretly.

Troublesome questions arise, of course, regarding personal competence, mental illness, and the definition of "voluntary." They are, however, no more difficult than those the courts and legislatures have been struggling with for a long time. The question finally is how far the state is willing to go to prevent people from exercising their choice to die. How much suffering are we willing to impose on people to negate their choices, and how far will we go to force them to submit to the will of the state in a show of power? I do not pretend answers are available that any of us can be fully comfortable with. I fear the tyrannical power of the government as much as I fear the excesses of individual freedom. I repeat, however, that we must do everything within our power to nourish in all people the desire to live and make suicide a far worse choice than living.

The variety of individual circumstances in which a person might choose to die rather than to go on is so wide-ranging and manifold that an exhaustive coverage is impossible. Suppose a person were badly burned all over and in constant excruciating pain, but recovery with good life prospects is ultimately likely. One might within hard-to-define limits reasonably resist the pleas of the person to be killed to obtain immediate release. How far one would go depends on the circumstances, and we shudder in horror at the prospect of having to confront the problem for ourselves or someone we love dearly. Remember the case of Dax Cowart. Likewise, in the case of mental illness or depression, perplexing choices arise as to what extreme we should go forcibly to prevent suicide in the long-term best interest of the patient. Every possible effort through counseling and medication should be made to make life tolerable if not desirable for every person. But that suicide should always be prevented by whatever means are necessary seems as cruel and inhumane as the decision to do nothing would be callous and uncaring. We are fallible and nearly helpless in the face of some dilemmas. We can only do the best we can with love, mercy, and compassion as our guide.

Further Reflections

The slippery-slope argument seems to assume that just beneath the surface are dangerous impulses so powerful that if we make a small move to legalize assistance in dying, all restraints will fall away. Sooner or later all sorts of people will want to kill themselves or do away with the most vulnerable among us who need special or expensive care or who are just inconvenient to bother with. I don't believe it. With few exceptions, everyone loves life, appreciates it, and wants to preserve it for themselves as long as any possibility of tolerable, hopeful existence remains. No intelligent, sane, moral person desires to force involuntary death on the innocent or to manipulate the dying to choose death, even if doing so would be convenient or save money.

In the last analysis, I think that the analogy of the slippery slope is basically wrong. We are not at the top of a hill so that the slightest nudge of the boulder will start it downward into an abyss. It feels more like we are near the bottom of a steep incline trying to push a boulder upward a few inches. The notion that success in moving the stone slightly suddenly creates a downward slope that cannot be resisted does not make sense. The implication seems to be that once we legalize assisted death, we lose our power of choice and some irresistible process takes over that inevitably propels us into disaster.

To be fair, let us observe that a few needed steps up the hill have been taken as compared to three or four decades ago in which the right to refuse treatment had not been firmly established. First we recognized that in certain desperate circumstances, patients or their legal proxies had a right to order the removal of life-sustaining treatment. Initially that included ventilators and only later was extended to hydration and nutrition. Even some opponents of assisted suicide who make the slippery-slope argument agree that these moves were justified. They just think we should not go any further. It can certainly be argued, however, that permitting assisted death in some circumstances is a reasonable next step that is in harmony with the moves that have already been made during the last few decades. All agree that we must draw lines somewhere. But where? That, we must keep repeating, is what the decisive debate is about.

Society has a choice at every step. Unless our citizens have the virtue, compassion, and good sense to know where to draw the line and enough realism to be on guard against abuses, we are in trouble anyway. In every area of life we have to make distinctions and sort out differences between one situation and another. We have to learn how to make decisions in the light of all the relevant factors that pertain to particular cases. Juries and judges are compelled to do this repeatedly. The same need for wisdom, discernment, and good judgment in relating principles to a diversity of circumstances holds for this issue.

One consideration does make me hesitant. It is not that once assisted suicide or voluntary active euthanasia is legalized under the most restrictive conditions, we will be inevitably driven by the force of logic or sheer momentum into unacceptable extremes. It is rather the baffling problems involved in having to make decisions in a multitude of circumstances that would bewilder the most discerning and compassionate minds and hearts. Situations would arise replete with such complexities, ambiguities, conflicting values, uncertainties, and relativities that the line between going far enough and going too far would be extremely difficult to draw. Incompetent administration of the rules, the possibility of error, and the likelihood of injustices springing from a failure of judgment and abuses originating from malice would further complicate the matter. Added to all this is the special vulnerability of the poor, minorities, the elderly, and the disabled to abuses related to money, prejudice, and sheer irresponsibility. Having a general rule against all assisted suicide and administered death is a way of avoiding these baffling and irresolvable problems. It is better, opponents maintain, not even to get into these murky areas. This is why we must never make it possible for people to have assistance in dying, even if in some particularly extreme circumstances it might be justified. While I am attracted to that option, I reject it. First of all, even if we grant the need for general rules, as I do, what are those rules to be? In the second place, we have to decide if general rules are to have exceptions. Not to allow exceptions may create injustices for some to whom the general rule does not apply. The reason we allow judges sometimes and juries at other times to have discretion in making judgments is to take into account exceptional circumstances that require a specific judgment in the application of general laws. On the other hand, a general rule is implicit in every decision made in particular circumstances. We are never quite done with the process of finding general rules to which we make no exceptions and making general rules that do allow exceptions. Our task is always to find the best rules and to define justifiable exceptions and then to devise a process for judging in particular cases and for making emendations. Making rules and allowing exceptions is a complicated, imperfect process subject to the limitations of human reasoning and fallible procedures.

All these considerations almost persuade me that it would be better to forbid any deliberate taking of life even when requested by a mentally competent, terminally-ill patient in unmanageable misery already at death's door. Some maintain that only a very few of those persons who request assistance in dying meet these requirements anyway. Most people who consider suicide are not near death, are not in immediate physical pain, and may not even have a terminal illness. Life has become intolerable, or so they think, because of depression or anxiety or other life circumstances that have created a sense of utter despair. Let us note, first of all, that this is a statistical point, not a moral one. Just because only a few meet the most stringent requirements that have been laid down does not mean that they should be denied the privilege of requesting assistance to make their imminent death easier.

However, the fact that most people who contemplate suicide are not near death does raise the terribly difficult question of how far this privilege should be extended. I refrain from abandoning the cause only because to admit the difficulty is merely to acknowledge that decisions in this area of life are no different from what we unavoidably face with respect to a horde of other problems. Life is filled with perplexing choices. To seek to avoid them in the cases of assisted dying is not a mark of prudence. Wisdom urges us to be circumspect, not to flee from responsibility. Avoidance is impossible anyway, since legislatures and the courts are already deeply involved. Let us grant that we deal here literally with life and death. Moreover, firm lines have to be drawn somewhere. But it is not at all self-evident that to deny the possibility of assisted death absolutely regardless of circumstances is the course that makes most rational and moral sense.

Let us agree that often when we draw a line, it is arbitrary and relative and not clear-cut or absolute. If we are to have the death penalty, exactly what crimes warrant execution? A simple example will further the point. At the very beginning of my career, I was teaching a college course in which I based the final grade on the average of five exams. Any numerical grade of 90.0 or above merited an A. The average for one student came out 89.9. At first, I concluded that I could not deny an A on such a small margin. Upon reflection, however, I realized that if I gave an A for 89.9, the next grade might come out 89.8. What was I to do then? It occurred to me that, as fine a point as it was, it was best to draw an absolute line between 90.0 and anything that fell short of that, no matter how small the margin. That resolved the issue, and I went about my business without worrying about being unfair to those who were almost there but not quite. Lines do have to be drawn somewhere. My argument is simply that it is not at all clear that where we draw that line now with regard to assisted death is where it ought to be drawn once and for all.

One final comment can end this section. The assumption seems to be not only that the slippery slope propels us onward to ever wider extensions of the right to choose death, but also that once having taken a step, we cannot go back. This is patently false. We once tried prohibition and later decided it did not work. Capital punishment has been on and then off and then back on the books in a number of states. Every policy choice can be rescinded if experience and deeper insight demand it. Given this fact, the fear of making a small warranted move now because of what might happen later is unfounded. Ultimately, slippery-slope arguments with respect to voluntary suicide rest on a deeper distrust of the capacity of society to make responsible judgments in the long run or to correct errors of policy when they become apparent. If this skepticism is well-founded, we are doomed anyway, slippery slopes or not. Slippery-slope arguments are not always wrong, but neither are they always valid. Care must be taken in every particular instance to separate insight from error, wisdom from folly, and caution from the groundless scare tactics of overzealous opponents.

The following chapter will take up two of the most contested and difficult issues in the current debate. Is there a moral difference between letting death happen and causing it? Is there a moral difference between intending only to relieve suffering despite hastening death and intending to cause death in order to relieve suffering?

Chapter 6

The Heart Of The Debate: Two Difficult Issues

Once we get past the controversy over slippery slopes, we come upon the two most difficult moral issues currently being debated. Physicians, lawyers, philosophers, and theologians are found on both sides. The position one holds depends on whether certain distinctions are regarded as logically, legally, medically, and morally crucial. We will see two instances in which opponents of assisted suicide find clear-cut points at which a bright line should be drawn. It is where the line is currently drawn. Our task will be to determine if this is where it ought to be drawn. To the heart of the moral debate we now turn.

Letting Death Happen And Causing It

A major argument against assisted dying relates to the distinction between letting death occur and intentionally causing death to happen. The claim is that a crucial moral difference exists between ceasing or withholding life support in irreversible cases and taking active steps that deliberately hasten death.[1] The reasoning is that when a patient who is fatally ill refuses life-sustaining treatment, death results from the underlying disease or condition, but if a patient is given lethal medication prescribed by a doctor, death is caused by the drug itself. Moreover, terminating treatment involves no intent to cause death but simply recognizes that the situation is hopeless and that medical science has done all it can do.

While accepted by eminent authorities in law, medicine, and ethics, the reasoning involved here, in my opinion, is spurious. In a set of circumstances in which the occurrence of death involves more than a single vital factor, to isolate one and call it the real or sole cause of death is bad logic. Whether one has removed life support or provided lethal medicine, the death occurs most immediately, directly, and sooner because of that specific act. Recently the Second and Ninth Circuit Courts rightly noted that withdrawing life-sustaining treatment is no less an act of killing than administering a lethal dose of medicine. Moreover, a positive human action is involved. Someone does something, that is, either removes a life-support system or provides lethal medicine. Moreover, an underlying terminal disease or some intolerable human circumstance is involved in both cases. A request for assistance in hastening the end of life would not be made if it were not. Human choice and agency are involved either way, and the result is a quicker death than otherwise would be the case.

Furthermore, the quicker death is often desired by patient, doctor, and family. The quicker, desired death is exactly the outcome of providing or administering lethal medicine. Dr. Leonard J. Deftos speaks of the legal irrelevance and moral ambiguity of the distinctions between active and passive procedures and adds that

> *such rumination about these categories is a physician-oriented and hospital-based exercise that overlooks the seminal fact that all serve the same intent* of the patient — *to choose and hasten the time of one's death.*[2]

Some critics protest, however, that when life-sustaining treatment is withdrawn, the patient would not die unless an underlying lethal pathology were present.[3] In the case of assisted suicide, the medicine kills on its own, whether or not a terminal illness exists. Perhaps so, but this objection misses the crucial point. In this connection Dr. David Orentlicher comments as follows:

> *If I entered an intensive care unit and shut off every patient's ventilator, I would be charged with the murder of every patient who died. It would be no defense that the patients' deaths were caused by their underlying illnesses. It is true that I would have acted without the patient's consent, but consent does not change the cause of a patient's death. The issue, then, is not whether*

assisted suicide causes death but whether it is a justifiable way to cause death.[4]

Furthermore, let us notice that while the right to refuse life-sustaining treatment is well established today, it was not always that clear. In 1976 the parents of Karen Ann Quinlan had to get an order from the New Jersey Supreme Court before doctors were allowed to remove her ventilator. In 1983 in the Barber case in California, two physicians were taken to court because they took away life-supporting treatment at the request of the family. An appellate court finally eliminated the murder charges.[5] The point is that once it was widely thought that taking away life-sustaining equipment was the immediate cause of death and thus should not be permitted. It is simply that now we believe it should be permitted. We think so today, not because it is not the immediate cause of death, but because it is justifiable under the circumstances. Now it is widely recognized that it is lawful killing. It is only a small move from that to recognize that under the same set of circumstances, assisted suicide may also be regarded as lawful killing.

Other arguments are made that upon close examination do not hold up.[6] It is argued that refusal of treatment is a negative right to be left alone, whereas assisted dying involves a positive right for aid. It is not that simple. Proponents argue that if a doctor and patient decide that help in dying is warranted, the state should leave them alone and not interfere with that choice. This is also a kind of negative right — the right to be left alone to carry out one's own choice. In similar fashion, it is argued that traditionally the law has recognized a right to be free of unwelcome intrusion upon the body. Hence, refusal of treatment is acceptable. To deny assistance to the dying forces nothing on the patient and thus no right is denied. Here again the protest misfires. States sometimes do force treatment upon people, for tuberculosis, for example. Courts have ordered pregnant women to accept treatment that would benefit them and the fetus. We recognize a right for emergency medical care. Again, it must be repeatedly emphasized that the crucial issue does not depend on fine distinctions between one thing and another or even on what is done or not done, but whether the actions that are taken are justified under the circumstances. Is a course of action the best for a particular situation, that is, better than the available alternatives, all things considered? It is on this question that our moral debate must be centered in the search of wisdom.

Yale Kamisar rightly argues that a society that prohibited patients from refusing life-sustaining treatment would be an unpleasant place to live and die.[7] We would be at the mercy of every technological advance. But could we not with equal cogency maintain that a society that denies assistance in dying to a hopelessly ill patient, thus condemning that person to live in intolerable misery until death naturally comes, is also not a good place to live?

Daniel Callahan and Kamisar correctly point out that removing life-sustaining treatment does not intend the patient's death or imply that the patient would be better off dead. Kamisar protests that if he stopped shoveling snow in a heavy storm because he could no longer keep up with it, it would not mean that he intended a driveway deep in snow. Likewise, to cease futile treatment does not aim to kill a patient but only recognizes that medical science has reached its limits and cannot be of any further assistance. While death follows more quickly, that is not the intent but only recognizes that it cannot be prevented. Assisted dying, on the other hand, does intend the patient's death. True enough, but that still leaves open the question as to whether the intention to cause death by deliberate action is justified by the fact that ending suffering sometimes takes priority over extending life.

Dr. David Orentlicher maintains that previously the law has drawn a bright line between the right of patients to refuse treatment and assisted suicide not because of any morally or logically sound differences between the two, but because the distinction provided a useful and usually good rule for distinguishing between morally valid and morally invalid decisions by patients to end their lives. We need general rules like this, he reasons, since a case by case determination would be too complicated and difficult. This particular distinction has worked well in general as a substitute for deciding individual cases. This is so because typically the demand for the withdrawal of life support has been made by people who were terminally ill and without much life worth living left no matter what was done or not done. The typical suicide we think of as not having that kind of justification.

However, the right to refuse treatment has been extended to include almost any patient and almost any treatment. Because of medical advances some terminally ill persons are in intractable pain but not on life-support systems. Under present law these people who desire to end their lives are prohibited from doing so. Yet the medical reasons for requesting assistance in dying are similar to those that originally led to the right of patients to refuse life-sustaining procedures. For this reason, he argues, the law is now changing to bring practice more in line with the moral reasoning of society.

Orentlicher offers a telling example.[8] Consider a 28-year-old who is despondent because of the recent breakup of a love affair and who temporarily requires a ventilator because of an acute asthma attack. The other person is 82 years old, suffers great and intractable pain from extensive metastatic cancer, and has only a few weeks to live. Under prevailing law the young person has a right to demand withdrawal of the ventilator, but the old person does not have a right to assisted suicide. Yet in terms of the reasons we allow people to refuse life-sustaining treatment, it would be more reasonable to refuse the request of the 28-year-old and to grant the request of the 82-year-old. The old man has not much life left not matter what we do, and hastening his desired death would relieve his agony. The young man has potentially many more years of good life and will doubtless in time get over his romantic disappointments and once more value his life. Ideally, we would grant some requests for help in committing suicide and some requests to withdraw treatment and deny others. If we are not willing to devise procedures for proceeding on a case by case basis, we need new general rules to serve as a normally-useful guide. Orentlicher argues that new rules are coming into practice through legislatures and the courts that recognize that medical condition is the crucial factor, not whether death results immediately from treatment withdrawal or by an assisted suicide. The point is that it is context and circumstance that determine what is morally appropriate.

Hence, while the distinction between passive and active euthanasia has a kind of surface appeal and logic, deeper analysis reveals it to be non-decisive. A difference of a sort exists between withdrawing treatment and assisted suicide. However, I deny that the difference is conclusive in determining what is morally permitted or mandated. The proper question is: What is the best thing that can be done under the circumstances when no alternative is desirable? We get our answer by determining what values and obligations are paramount and what the consequences of various actions will be. In some instances the best of ambiguous choices is to hasten death by deliberate means for those who choose that alternative or when proxies act for an unconscious or incompetent patient.

Suppose an infant is born with multiple disabilities so severe that the only prospect is to engage in a series of painful, invasive procedures that are highly unlikely to succeed. The parents decide against treatment. Is it better to put the child aside and provide comfort care until death comes or to hasten death mercifully by deliberate action? Imagine a young person who has been in a coma for years with no reason to believe that recovery will ever occur, but with artificial hydration and nutrition could live indefinitely. If the life support systems are removed at the request of authorized proxies, should the patient be allowed to die slowly or quickly terminated by a lethal injection? When compassion is the only motive in all involved, I fail to see the moral superiority of letting die over causing death in these cases.

The literature is filled with subtle and profound discussions of what is the true cause of death, as if this would resolve the moral issues. Since we are obligated not only to do no harm but also to do good, the issue turns on motivations, the values expressed, the obligations lived out, the nature of the acts, and their consequences. Declarations that we are guilty of wrong if we are the direct and immediate cause of death but innocent if nature, disease, or the condition is the underlying cause miss the main point. If death is hastened, whether (1) by lethal injection or (2) by withdrawing life-sustaining treatment, then human choice and agency are implicated in shortening life in both instances. The relative degree of human causation is secondary to more fundamental factors of motivation, the values expressed, and the consequences.

Relieving Suffering And Causing Death

Another claim made by opponents of physician-assisted and physician-administered death is that it is permissible to give massive doses of pain medicine to dying patients if the intent is to relieve suffering even though the unavoidable consequence is to quicken death. But it is wrong to do exactly the same thing if the intent is to cause death more quickly in order to relieve unnecessary, pointless suffering. It all depends on the motive, according to the theory of the "double effect." The first rejoinder is that motive alone is not the sole determinant of morality. The nature of the act and the consequences count too. Imagine someone who burns down a barn to kill the rats who were rapidly eating the corn. We would not be impressed with the claim that this act was justified because the sole aim was to kill the rats and not to destroy the barn and the corn. The point of this absurd example is that both effects matter and must be evaluated, not only the intended one. In cases in which death is going to occur soon no matter what we do, hastening death by administering pain medicine may be warranted by the relief of suffering that results. Why not admit that the pain medicine is given to accomplish both effects, if that is the patient's choice? Only a very fine line separates that from deliberately administering a drug that causes death quickly in order to relieve pointless, excruciating suffering.

The line gets even finer when the only way to relieve suffering is to administer anesthetic levels of medication that keep the patient in a deep sleep-like state until death comes. As Dr. Leonard Deftos notes:

> ... *the legally and medically accepted practice of "terminal sedation" in fact comes closer to forbidden euthanasia than does assisted suicide, since it is the physician, not the patient, who administers the drug of death. So any line between the voluntariness and involuntariness of physician assistance in suicide has*

already been crossed by current medical, legal, and even ethical canons. And it is physicians who have crossed the line.[9]

Putting all this together, we have four possibilities:
1. giving pain medicine to relieve suffering despite the fact that it hastens death,
2. providing continuous anesthetic levels of medicine and thus terminal sedation to relieve suffering until death occurs,
3. giving pain medicine in order to relieve pain and to hasten death, and
4. administering a lethal injection that causes death quickly in order to relieve suffering.

Moral reasoning that permits 1 and 2 if the sole motive is to relieve suffering but forbids 3 and 4 because the intent includes the deliberate hastening of death is spurious in my opinion. The objective result is the same, except that in 4 death might mercifully come a little sooner. Instances may arise in which it may be preferable to end suffering by causing death rather than to extend life slightly at the cost of immense, needless agony. In any case, the decision in these circumstances should be made on the basis of how the value of extending life is weighed against the value of relieving suffering, not on motive alone when the "double effect" cannot be avoided.

That leads me to the second response. To permit the administration of pain medicine in order to relieve suffering even though it hastens death gives the case away. It does so because the principle of that action is that in some instances relieving suffering is preferable to extending life a little bit longer. That is exactly the principle for which I am contending. If extending life even a little bit always takes absolute precedence over relieving suffering, one could not administer medicine to relieve even the most excruciating pain if it hastens death even slightly. If it does not always take absolute precedence, then it becomes a relative value to be weighed against others. That is my contention, and I have expressed the view that sometimes ending suffering takes priority over extending life. Once that judgment is made, we will no longer worry about "double effects" purified by intent or the distinction between letting death happen and causing it to happen.

Finally, let us observe that even if one provides or administers medicine that one knows full well will end the life of the patient, one can still claim that the intent was not to kill but to relieve suffering. Dr. Jack Kevorkian has repeatedly defended himself in court by claiming that his purpose was to relieve suffering, not to kill, even though his procedures were lethal in outcome. All this means is that moral issues cannot be settled by reference to intent alone. Objectively and ethically speaking, does it matter decisively whether one's subjective intent is to relieve suffering by killing or to relieve suffering despite unfortunately killing? I am not contending that motives are unimportant or irrelevant, but only that it is one of several factors that have to be taken into consideration, not the sole determinant of right and wrong.

This concludes the analysis of the issues. In the next chapter I will offer a brief historical review and make some proposals about where we go from here.

---

1. This distinction was invoked by the Supreme Court decision of June 26, 1997. Chief Justice Rehnquist, writing the unanimous decision in the case of *Vacco v. Quill* in which the Court held that New York's prohibition of assisting suicide does not violate the Equal Protection Clause of the Constitution, wrote:

   > The distinction comports with fundamental legal principles of causation and intent. First, when a patient refuses life sustaining medical treatment, he dies from an underlying fatal disease or pathology; but if a patient ingests lethal medication prescribed by a physician, he is killed by that medication.

2. Leonard J. Deftos, "Physician Assistance in Dying," *Postgraduate Medicine* (June 1997).

3. Daniel Callahan, "When Self-Determination Runs Amok," *Hastings Center Report*, 1992, vol. 22. no. 2, 52-5, and E. D. Pellegrino, "Doctors Must Not Kill," *Journal of Clinical Ethics*, 1992, no. 3, 95-102.

4. David Orentlicher, "The Legalization of Physician-Assisted Suicide," *The New England Journal of Medicine*, Vol. 335, No. 9 (August 29, 1996).

5. See Orentlicher, "The Legalization of Physician-Assisted Suicide," for both of these cases.

6. In this section I am much indebted to Dr. David Orentlicher for his insights. See note 4.

7. Yale Kamisar, "Against Assisted Suicide — Even in a Very Limited Form," Testimony to the Committee on the Judiciary, United States House of Representatives, April 29, 1996.

8. Orentlicher, "The Legalization of Physician-Assisted Suicide."

9. Deftos, "Physician Assistance in Dying."

Chapter 7

Where We Are And A Suggestion

The issues have been laid out and the arguments for and against assisted suicide and administered death have been analyzed. I have set forth my own conclusions and offered the reasoning that led to them. This final chapter offers a brief review of developments during the last quarter of a century that have brought us to the present and to the issues that dominate the debate as we approach the end of this millennium. I will offer some proposals about next steps that would be helpful. Finally, I will argue that the moral and legal issues raised in this essay ultimately point to a religious resolution that law, medicine, morality, and human choice cannot provide.

Legal And Moral Developments

In the last quarter of a century the rights of people to have a say in their medical treatment have been extended considerably. This has involved a series of court decisions that reflect a change of thinking among the general population. In 1970 the right of a patient to refuse treatment was not firmly established. In 1973 Dax Cowart was badly burned over two-thirds of his body in a propane gas explosion. For fourteen months he remained in a hospital and fought against treatment and begged to be allowed and assisted to die. But he was treated against his will. He survived the ordeal and later achieved success and happiness in life. However, he dedicated himself to the promotion of patients' rights. While he is glad to be alive, he still thinks he should not have been treated without his consent. His ordeal raised the subject of forced treatment in a forceful way. As late as 1983 in the Barber case in California, two doctors were prosecuted for removing life-sustaining procedures at the request of the family, but a higher court ordered the murder charges dropped.[1]

Change, however, was underway. Karen Ann Quinlan had existed for months in a persistent vegetative state. In 1976 in a landmark case the New Jersey Supreme Court gave permission for her ventilator to be removed at the request of her parents. However, no petition was made for the removal of a feeding tube, and it remained. She actually lived for another ten years sustained by the nasogastric tube that supplied nutrition but without the ventilator. Says Dr. Leonard Deftos about this situation:

> *Prior to this case, such medical decisions were often made with pietistic and paternalistic attitudes by courts and physicians. Concerned about possible prosecution and probable censure, physicians imposed life-sustaining machines and procedures on their patients, even against their will. Courts sometimes mercifully intervened, but often belatedly.*[2]

By the late 1980s the distinction previously honored between respirators and feeding tubes was disappearing. In 1986 in the Elizabeth Bouvia case, a California Court of Appeals overturned the ruling of the lower court and ordered that the feeding tube be removed. Without hydration and food, she would die. In 1990 in the Nancy Cruzan case, the Supreme Court of the United States rendered a decision that saw no hindrance in the fact that the life-sustaining equipment in her case was a feeding tube. When the case went back to Missouri for a final verdict, the state court ordered that the tube in her stomach that provided hydration and nutrition be removed. She died within a few days.

The other side of the right to refuse treatment is the right to demand treatment. Does a patient or family have the legal prerogative to insist on treatment in situations that are regarded by medical professionals as futile and inappropriate? One recent case illustrates the point. Baby K was an infant born in 1992 with anencephaly in a hospital in Virginia. Anencephalic babies are born with most of their brain missing. Generally, they are provided comfort care only. In this instance the mother demanded aggressive treatment. The doctor in charge of Baby K's care believed that to do what the mother requested was unwise. It was futile and improper. The doctor refused to comply and asked a federal court for a judgment. The court by a narrow margin ruled that the hospital could not deny emergency treatment.[3] Should decisions like this remain in the hands of parents, regardless of what physicians think? Has patient autonomy gone too far when the treatment insisted on is useless and unsuitable? Should limits be put on what patients or their families can demand?

The right to refuse treatment even if death results, however, is now well established in law, practice, and in general acceptance of citizens. This legal guarantee has been incorporated into state laws, and legislatures have created living wills, advanced directives, and durable powers of attorney. In 1990 Congress passed the Patient Self-Determination Act. All these measures have extended personal autonomy by allowing people to state in advance their wishes regarding life-sustaining equipment. Hospitals and nursing homes allow patients to sign a "do not resuscitate order," which, as Dr. Leonard Deftos notes, is a way of choosing to hasten death.

However, the distinction between withdrawing life-preserving treatment and assisted suicide has persisted in legal and medical ethics. That difference has long been questioned by some theologians, lawyers, philosophers, doctors, and medical ethicists. An important article by my former student James Rachels in 1975 became the focus of much discussion. Rachels argued persuasively that the distinction between passive and active euthanasia is not crucial for medical ethics.[4] Some courts have now rejected it. In April 1996 the Second Circuit Court in *Quill v. Vacco* concluded that the ending of life by withdrawal of life support is in fact a form of assisted suicide. An act is performed in removing the equipment, and life is shortened. Hence, the state cannot grant a right to refuse life-sustaining treatment but forbid equal consideration to those who choose to die by lethal drugs, since both are in fact forms of suicide. The court concluded that New York's prohibition of assisted suicide is a violation of the Equal Protection provision of the Constitution. In March 1996 the Ninth Circuit in *Washington v. Glucksberg* referred to the Cruzan case and noted that without the feeding tube that was removed by court order, she would die. Hence, this decision necessarily implies a liberty interest in hastening death, that is, committing suicide by starvation. The court concluded that Washington's prohibition against aiding someone to hasten death is a violation of the Due Process provision of the Constitution. We have a right to choose the time and manner of our death.

Here we need to note that both the Second and the Ninth Circuit Courts strictly speaking found a right to assisted suicide in which the physician only provides the means or medication. The patient actually performs the deed that leads to death. The Second Circuit Court specifically distinguishes assisted suicide from euthanasia in which the physician administers the drug that kills. Euthanasia, the court noted, is murder according to New York law. The Ninth Circuit Court was not so strict. Judge Stephen Reinhardt acknowledged that in a future case it might be difficult to find a principled difference between physician-assisted suicide and physician-administered death. He concluded that it was less important who administers the lethal medicine than who determines whether the person's life shall end.

This is where matters stood when the Supreme Court heard these two cases in 1997. The debate now centers around whether a decisive legal, medical, and moral difference exists between withholding or withdrawing life-sustaining treatment (including both respirators and feeding tubes) and assisted suicide. The former is now established in law, practice, ethical theory, and general acceptance by the public. The latter is the point around which controversy rages. Some, like Yale Kamisar, argue that a bright line should be drawn between ceasing treatment and assisted suicide. If we cross this line, we put ourselves on a slippery slope that leads to disastrous extensions of the right to choose death. Others, like David Orentlicher and Leonard Deftos, see assisted suicide as a reasonable extension of rights based on the same principles that justify the liberty to refuse treatment that has been established in law and practice during the last quarter of a century. Throughout this essay, I have sided with Orentlicher and Deftos against Kamisar.

On June 26, 1997, the Supreme Court made a unanimous decision stating that the Constitution upholds the right of a state to forbid assisted suicide. In *Washington v. Glucksberg* the Court held that Washington's prohibition against causing or aiding a suicide does not violate the Due Process clause. In *Vacco v. Quill* the Court held that New York's prohibition against assisted suicide does not violate the Equal Protection clause. The effect was to deny that the Constitution establishes a right to assistance in ending one's life.

One immediate implication of the Court decision agreed to by all parties is that new and more effective steps must be taken to ensure that the best possible care of the dying is provided. The goal would be that, because life continues to be desirable or at least tolerable, the request for help in dying would not arise. This is presently not possible in every case. That is why, in extreme situations when a quick death is preferable to prolonged dying in agony, assisted suicide should be legalized.

Reports indicate that many patients do not receive maximum relief of pain and suffering. No excuse can be given for the failure of doctors to provide the greatest alleviation of pain and suffering that current medicine is capable of. Fortunately, awareness of the need to provide better care of the dying is increasing. Opponents of assisted suicide express fear that the poor, the disabled, and the marginalized might be put under pressure to end their lives if doctors were legally allowed to hasten death. Then let them, and all of us, demand that society and doctors find ways to provide for every dying patient and for everyone who requires long-term care the most effective relief of suffering that contemporary medical science has at its disposal.

It must be stressed that care does not mean simply treating illness and pain medically with the most advanced and effective means but includes attention to the whole person. Patients need love, companionship, a sense of control, and the capacity to retain their dignity. They should be dealt with as suffering human beings and not as objects to be managed efficiently with drugs, tests, and technical procedures. In the presence of the ultimate issues of life and death, we need trained medical professionals with heart and not simply with medical knowledge and technical skills. What does it profit us if the body is treated with the latest and best that science and technology have to offer if our spirits are denied the loving support of family, doctors, and a compassionate society? Attention to the whole person can keep alive the desire to live and sometimes result in a change of mind about wanting to die. In Georgia Larry McAfee was left a quadriplegic after a motorcycle accident and got a court order to disconnect the ventilator that kept him alive. He decided he wanted to live after all when wide publicity about his case brought forth support of people and services that made him value his life.[5]

The debate will go on. A 1997 CNN/*USA Today* poll indicated that 55 percent of people are in favor of physician-assisted suicide, while only 37 percent express opposition. Other polls in recent years have yielded similar results. A newspaper poll in upstate New York found that 63 percent of citizens and 59 percent of physicians favored physician-assisted suicide.[6] An AMA opinion survey in 1995 found that 55 percent of the public and 63 percent of physicians favored physician-assisted suicide under some conditions. The same survey showed that 54 percent of the public and 56 percent of physicians would approve a physician's administering medicines to cause death under certain conditions.[7] The Supreme Court did not rule out the possibility that individual states might legalize assisted suicide. It only concluded that it is constitutional to prohibit it. Hence, the new battleground moves to each of the states.

In 1994 voters in Oregon voted to allow to physicians to prescribe lethal medicines. After a series of court battles opponents persuaded the legislature to put the measure on the ballot once more. On November 4, 1997, by the margin of 60 percent to 40 percent the citizens voted to keep the law. Legislation in late 1997 was pending in eight states: Hawaii, Illinois, Maine, Massachusetts, Michigan, Vermont, Washington, and Wisconsin. Michigan, South Carolina, Illinois, and Vermont also had bills before them that would ban assisted suicide.[8]

A Suggestion

Given the importance of the issue and the wisdom of proceeding cautiously, I propose the following in light of the Supreme Court decision of June 26, 1997. Let some forward-looking states legalize physician assistance in dying under very restricted conditions.

(1) The patient must be hopelessly ill and near death, (2) mentally competent, (3) in great and uncontrollable misery, and (4) make a voluntary, persisting request to be given assistance in hastening death. The law should require confirmation of all these conditions by appropriate means.

The several states could devise their own procedures, so that many options might be tried and evaluated. Let us then have an extensive period of experimentation to determine what actually occurs when assisted suicide is legalized under these strictly limited conditions. Meanwhile, the issues should be widely discussed by a variety of citizens from all walks of life in light of all the facts that become available from the various experiments. Only then should any consideration be given to whether the circumstances under which persons may request assistance in dying should be broadened and, if so, in what circumstances. Only by actual experimentation of our own can we know what would actually occur in this country, how many people would be involved, what the consequences would be for physicians, the families of patients, and others. Both sides appeal to the experience of the Netherlands with assisted suicide to support their own views. Assisted suicide there is not legal but simply is not prosecuted when certain rules are followed. What happens in other countries may be instructive in its own right, but it does not necessarily indicate what would happen in the United States. If, after thorough evaluation, a majority of citizens are convinced that any step taken was a mistake, the legislation could be rescinded.

From the outset I have acknowledged that in principle, I am willing to go further than this modest proposal goes. For now I am only arguing that we should take this small step forward to legalize assisted suicide. Were my proposal to become law, I might change my mind in the future on the basis on what actually happens when it is tested in real life. I might even agree that we should rescind even that small move and prohibit it altogether. I do not fear that my proposal puts us on a disastrous slippery slope for reasons I have outlined at length. If there is a slippery slope, we are already on it. We got on it when we decided that we should not always do everything in our power to keep dying patients alive absolutely as long as humanly possible using every means available. We are already several steps from that, and most people agree that they should have been taken. The question now as always is where to draw the line.

I do agree that when the patient is conscious, the case is strongest when she or he is competent, dying soon anyway no matter what we do or do not do, is suffering intolerably without possible relief, and voluntarily requests a quick death with assistance. The further we move away from these conditions, the weaker the case gets. But where we should draw the line is not conclusive and demonstrable on the basis of what we know now.

James Rachels has made an alternative proposal that is also worthy of consideration. His suggestion is that mercy killing be made acceptable by law as a defense against murder.[9] This move would parallel the status of self-defense as a justification for taking the life of another. If the defense could show that the killing was done upon the request of a terminally-ill patient undergoing great agony and that the act was done out of mercy in order to relieve suffering, the accused would be acquitted. The great merit of this proposal is that it avoids the difficult problem of having to write rules under which assisted suicide would be legal. It would not require a committee to decide when all the rules had been observed. Some situations are so complicated and so filled with uncertainty and ambiguity that providing adequate safeguards against abuse while defining conditions in which death could be deliberately hastened legally would be perplexing. This is a weighty factor in favor of the Rachels recommendation. The hazard is that the defense would have to convince a jury that a mercy killing had indeed taken place. This might be difficult given the circumstances. Some unfortunate person might be unjustly found guilty of murder by a skeptical jury or by some members on it who were so opposed to mercy killing that they simply would not vote for acquittal, no matter what the law said. Complicated and ambiguous cases would still arise that would test the wisdom of juries. Nevertheless, Rachels has made a proposal that states should consider along with the possibility of simply legalizing assisted suicide under certain well-defined and limited conditions. Many citizens in Canada have proposed moves along this line in the light of the trial of Robert Latimer for killing his twelve-year-old daughter with carbon monoxide. The Supreme Court decision of June 26, 1997, was a cautious one. It only concluded that no right to assisted suicide is provided in the Constitution. The effect was to throw the issue back to the states. Hence, I make these proposals as a judicious way to proceed with ample opportunity for citizens to participate in democratic processes to establish the will of the people.

My fear is that this problem will prove to be as polarizing as the abortion issue. The spectacle of citizens dividing up into warring camps, each confident that they alone possess the whole truth, is not a happy one. We do not need another issue in which partisans insist that their opponents are lacking in either decency or moral wisdom. Nevertheless, we must proceed in the hope that humility about our own views and respect for the integrity and insights of others will enable us to participate in a common search for moral discernment about problems that tax our reasoning capacities to their very utmost limit. At the same time I am realistic about the fact that bitter controversy probably lies ahead over the issue. We should be prepared for loud and passionate debates in which religious people confidently claim the authority of God for contradictory positions. Alas, this is the way it has always been. Calmer voices on all sides of the issue need to urge humility and openness on the part of everyone.

Final Reflections

A few days after the Supreme Court decision of June 1997, I received an e-mail message from someone whose mother had died recently after a prolonged period of unrelieved agony. She had the best care present-day medicine can provide, but her misery could not be alleviated. The story was powerful and heartbreaking. In their despair parent and child prayed for a quick death that would relieve the intolerable suffering that doctors could not manage. The writer was justifiably angry that the law did not allow steps to be taken that would have brought merciful relief by hastening the death that mother and family so earnestly desired. Since then I have received other messages from people with debilitating and life-threatening illnesses that are leading them to think about ways to end their suffering without putting those who assist them in jeopardy of prosecution. Stories like these provide the most powerful argument in favor of legalizing physician-assisted dying in extreme cases under carefully defined and limited circumstances with all necessary safeguards provided to prevent abuse.

Sometimes human beings confront limits to their wisdom. We make decisions in the presence of objective uncertainty and conflicting values. Tragedy and ambiguity pervade the scene. No decisions or legal arrangements are foolproof, infallible, or free from the possibility of abuse because of ill intent or despite good intentions. Sometimes every possible course of action makes us uneasy. Every available option will cause harm as well as accomplish something good. In these cases we simply have to act in obedience to the best we know up to now. We proceed in fear and trembling and with modesty about our wisdom and moral insight. And we can continue to subject our own convictions to the scrutiny of others whose criticism we trust in the hope that deeper insight will dawn regarding what love bids us do for each other when life becomes a burden rather than a blessing.

In some cases, conflicting values will create deep-rooted ambiguities and unavoidable tragedy. Such heartbreaking situations are not resolvable at the moral level but require religious resources of grace that mercifully release us from the otherwise unbearable burdens of our finitude and fallibility. In this regard I am a classical Protestant who finds the heart of the Good News in the proclamation that we are saved by grace through faith and not by our works. I think this includes our intellectual works in trying to reason about the right and the good. We are sinful, and we are finite. We are saved by grace not only from our moral failures but from the necessity of being infallible in the quest for truth. We can no more discover the perfect and whole truth about ultimate matters of existence and ethics than we can achieve moral perfection, although we are obligated to do our best in both the ethical and intellectual realms. We fail because we lack the moral will to do what we know is right, but we also confront baffling situations in which there are no unambiguous moral choices. We are limited by our own finitude and fallibility and by conflicting values in the objective situation. We can only hope to discover the lesser evil or the relatively better good. The alternatives to grace are utter despair over our inability to discover unambiguous moral truth or pretentious claims to absolute wisdom and ethical certainty not justified by the facts. Our final recourse is to the mercy of God, who has pity on us pathetic, error-prone creatures, who "knows our frame," who "remembers that we are dust" (Psalm 103:13-14 RSV).

---

1. *Barber v. Superior Court*, 195 Cal Rptr 484 (Ct App 1983).

2. Leonard J. Deftos, "Physician Assistance in Dying," *Postgraduate Medicine* (June 1997).

3. "Issues: Background on the Right to Die," *Choice in Dying* (Internet site, December 17, 1997).

4. James Rachels, "The Distinction Between Active Killing and Allowing to Die," *The New England Journal of Medicine* (January 9, 1975), 78-80.

5. David Orentlicher, "The Legalization of Physician-Assisted Suicide, *The New England Journal of Medicine* (August 29, 1996).

6. *Democrat and Chronicle*, Rochester, New York (November 6, 1997), 6A.

7. *The Park Ridge Center Bulletin* (September/October 1997), 13.

8. *Democrat and Chronicle*, Rochester, New York (November 6, 1997), 6A.

9. James Rachels, *The End of Life: Euthanasia and Morality* (New York: Oxford University Press, 1986).

Suggestions for Further Reading

The literature on assisted death is large and growing. I have included a few selected recent titles. The number of issues and arguments on suicide and euthanasia is limited. Hence, after looking at a few books, the reader will become familiar with the framework within which the debate is conducted. After that, further investigation will reveal mostly repetition, along with the peculiar style and outlook of individual authors.

Battin, Margaret Pabst. *The Death Debate: Ethical Issues in Suicide.* New York: Prentice-Hall, 1995.

_____. *The Least Worst Death: Essays in Bioethics on the End of Life.* New York: Oxford University Press, 1994.

Beauchamp, Tom L., and Childress, James F., editors. *Principles of Biomedical Ethics.* 4th ed. Oxford: Oxford University Press, 1994.

_____. *Ethical Issues in Death and Dying.* New York: Prentice-Hall, 1996.

_____, editor. *Intending Death: the Ethics of Assisted Suicide and Euthanasia.* Upper Saddle River, New Jersey: Prentice-Hall, 1996.

Hamel, Ronald P., and DuBose, Edwin R., editors. *Must We Suffer Our Way to Death?: Cultural and Theological Perspectives on Death by Choice.* Dallas: Southern Methodist University Press, 1996.

Hendin, Herbert. *Seduced by Death: Doctors, Patients and the Dutch Cure*. New York: W. W. Norton, 1996.

Hill, T. Patrick, and Shirley, David. *A Good Death: Taking More Control at the End of Your Life/Choice in Dying*. Reading, Massachusetts: Addison-Wesley Publishing Co., 1992.

Humber, James M., et. al., editors. *Physician-Assisted Death*. Totowa, New Jersey: Humana Press, 1994.

Humphrey, Derek, *Lawful Exit: the Limits of Freedom for Help in Dying*. Junction City, Oregon: Norris Lane Press, 1993.

Keown, John, editor. *Euthanasia Examined: Ethical, Clinical, and Legal Perspectives*. Cambridge: Cambridge University Press, 1995.

Long, Robert Emmet, editor. *Suicide*. New York: H. W. Wilson, 1995.

May, William F. *Testing the Medical Covenant: Active Euthanasia and Health Care Reform*. Grand Rapids, Michigan: Eerdmans, 1996.

Quill, Timothy. *Death and Dignity: Making Choices and Taking Charge*. New York: Norton, 1993.

_____. *Midwife Through the Dying Process*. Baltimore: Johns Hopkins University Press, 1996.

Rachels, James. *The End of Life: Euthanasia and Morality*. New York: Oxford University Press, 1986.

Smith, Wesley J. *Forced Exit: The Slippery Slope from Suicide to Legalized Murder*. New York: Random House, 1997.

Weir, Robert F., et. al. *Physician-Assisted Suicide*. Bloomington: Indiana University Press, 1997.

Urofsky, Melvin I., and Urofsky, Philip E., editors. *The Right to Die: a Two-Volume Anthology of Scholarly Articles*. New York: Garland Publishing, 1996.